Telemedicine in Orthopedic Surgery and Sports Medicine

T0171901

Alfred Atanda Jr.
John F. Lovejoy III
Editors

Telemedicine in Orthopedic Surgery and Sports Medicine

Development and Implementation in Practice

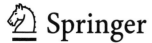 Springer

Editors
Alfred Atanda Jr.
Department of Orthopedic
Surgery
Nemours/Alfred I. duPont
Hospital for Children
Wilmington, DE
USA

John F. Lovejoy III
Department of Orthopaedics,
Sports Medicine and Physical
Medicine and Rehabilitation
University of Central Florida
School of Medicine, Nemours
Children's Hospital
Orlando, FL
USA

ISBN 978-3-030-53878-1   ISBN 978-3-030-53879-8   (eBook)
https://doi.org/10.1007/978-3-030-53879-8

This Springer imprint is published by the registered company Springer Nature Switzerland AG
The registered company address is: Gewerbestrasse 11, 6330 Cham, Switzerland

Preface

Today, electronic communication is embedded in the daily life of the majority of people throughout the world. Whether it is the text message to your family and friends, the multiple social media platforms that allow us to have a larger circle of influence, or the ability to schedule services and purchase goods, electronic communication is how the majority of people manage their lives. In the realm of medicine, the extension of this electronic provision of services has developed into what we know as telemedicine. As editors of this book, we have reflected on how we discovered telemedicine, and like many things in our careers, it was through a personal experience with a patient, that N of 1, that changed the course of our lives. To highlight this point is the story of Dr. Atanda and his patient Tom:

> In the summer of 2015, I had a patient, "Tom," who needed an anterior cruciate ligament reconstruction. He and his family lived near a popular beach destination about 100 miles from our hospital. In the recovery room after Tom's surgery, Tom's father told me how grateful the family felt for the care I had provided his son and that if I ever came down to the beach I should visit the family at the store they operated. It turned out, that a week later I was already planning to go to that beach with some friends. When I arrived at the beach, I visited Tom's family's store and chatted with his father. I had asked how Tom was doing and his father said that he was doing well, but was having some trouble with his post-operative knee brace. When I inquired further his father asked if I wouldn't mind calling Tom on the phone as he was at home recovering. While speaking with Tom, it was still a bit unclear as to the issue with the brace. Tom then suggested that we FaceTime so he could show me visually what was wrong. Once I could see his leg in the brace, I quickly understood the issue and we fixed it. I continued

to chat with Tom for another 5 minutes, inquiring how he was doing, how he rated his pain, and also had him point his camera so I could inspect his wound.

As I drove back from the beach, I suddenly appreciated how long a trip it was from their home to our hospital. It then dawned on me that Tom was scheduled to come back and see me for his first post-operative visit in just two days. I thought to myself, "What is he really going to get out of coming to see me in the office?" I had already seen his wound, watched him bend and extend his knee, talked to him about his pain and pain medication, and had seen that he was quite comfortable in his home environment. I immediately called Tom's father and told him that there was no need to come in-person for that first week post-operative visit and that we could see him at the three-week post-operative visit instead. And that was my first experience with Telemedicine................

Five years since this encounter, we have created a robust, nationally recognized orthopedic telemedicine program. We started with simple post-operative visits, added provider to provider consultations, linked virtual triage of new patients, created virtual athletic team coverage, and began offering second opinions. With support of our senior leadership, the telemedicine program has continuously evolved, constantly pushing the envelope, prototyping, failing, thinking, collaborating, and working tirelessly to re-imagine how orthopedic patients are triaged and evaluated throughout our healthcare ecosystem.

We hope this book will serve as a guide for orthopedic providers anywhere along the spectrum of their telemedicine journey. Whether you're still researching the right platform to initiate your program, trying to grow an existing platform, or using your platform for more advanced triage by connecting with an emergency room doctor half way around the world, this book will hopefully bring you closer to your goal. Remember that telemedicine is a tool, just like a reflex hammer or a stethoscope. It has to be used for the appropriate patient, by a provider that's comfortable using it, in the right clinical situation, at the right time. Telemedicine is not meant to replace traditional in-person care but rather to augment it. Today this is more apparent than ever, as although horrible and devastating, the COVID-19 pandemic of 2020 has brought the value and importance of telemedicine to the global stage. In such a crisis, telemedicine is a reliable and efficient way to keep patients, staff, and providers safe while maintaining high quality orthopedic care. Remember, though, whether it's to get through a crisis or to create a long-term digital health solution, it is important to do your homework before you implement telemedicine into your existing practice. Make sure to research state and federal guidelines, policies, and laws to ensure your program is in compliance with all applicable legal and licensing requirements. Regulatory compliance will also support your billing and payment structure as well. As with any new endeavor, you to have remain patient and flexible, as successful implementation and integration will not happen immediately. However, once your program is firmly established, we believe you will find telemedicine is a great way to stay relevant within the evolving healthcare landscape, provides convenient high-quality care, and will allow you to re-imagine how you deliver orthopedic care to your patients.

Wilmington, DE, USA   Alfred Atanda Jr.
Orlando, FL, USA   John F. Lovejoy III

Acknowledgments

First and foremost, I would like to thank Josh and Jonah, my two incredible sons for loving me and supporting me more than any father could ask for. I love you with all of my heart and I am so proud of both of you. It has been a tremendous pleasure to watch you grow up to be the fine young boys that you are today.

I would also like to thank the extended Atanda family. My mother Docia, my father Alfred Sr, and my six siblings Eric, Sylvia, Edward, Cynthia, Robert, and Korantemaa and the 20 Atanda grandchildren have been my inspiration, support system, and life companions. They've spent countless hours listening to me ramble on about telemedicine both in person and on my YouTube channel. They've loved, guided, and supported me my entire life and for that I will be forever grateful.

To my entire orthopedic and sports medicine family at Nemours, especially Ashley, Kaitlin, and Karen, you have taught me so much about myself and how to be a better person. You have supported and put up with me for almost 10 years now. I can't thank you enough for everything that you've done for my sports medicine career as well as my life in general. There is no "I" in team and I definitely couldn't have done any of this without you.

Lastly, I would like to thank John Lovejoy, Will Mackenzie, Carey Officer, Mary Lee, Pat Barth, Sue Voltz, Natalina Zisa, Joanne Murren-Boezem, Lisa Nichols, Melissa Sayles, Allison Micich, Sue Lindell, Jackie Sykes, Trent DeVore, Brad Way, and the entire Nemours organization for all of the support, encouragement, and love that they have showed me in my journey to become a better person, surgeon, and now author.

Contents

Contributors

Alfred Atanda Jr., MD Department of Orthopedic Surgery, Nemours/Alfred I. duPont Hospital for Children, Wilmington, DE, USA

Patrick Barth, MD Division of Otolaryngology, Department of Surgery, Nemours/Alfred I. duPont Hospital for Children, Wilmington, DE, USA

Jason Goldwater, MA, MPA Atlas Research, LLC, Washington, DC, USA

R. Michael Greiwe, MD Shoulder, Elbow and Sports Medicine, OrthoLive, CEO and OrthoCincy, Edgewood, KY, USA

Tina Gustin, DNP, CNS, RN Old Dominion University, Norfolk, VA, USA

Judd E. Hollander, MD Healthcare Delivery Innovation, Thomas Jefferson University, Philadelphia, PA, USA

Strategic Health Initiatives, Sidney Kimmel Medical College, Philadelphia, PA, USA

Finance and Healthcare Enterprises, Department of Emergency Medicine, Sidney Kimmel Medical College, Philadelphia, PA, USA

Betty A. Hovey, CCS-P, CPC, CDIP, CPMA, CPC-I Compliant Health Care Solutions, Lemont, IL, USA

John F. Lovejoy III, MD Department of Orthopaedics, Sports Medicine and Physical Medicine and Rehabilitation, University of Central Florida School of Medicine, Nemours Children's Hospital, Orlando, FL, USA

Amanda Martin, MHA Center for Rural Health Innovation, Spruce Pine, NC, USA

Joanne Murren-Boezem, MD Nemours Children's Health System, Center for Health Delivery Innovation, Orlando, FL, USA

Steve North, MD, MPH, FAAFP Center for Rural Health Innovation, Spruce Pine, NC, USA

Carey Officer, BS, Business Administration Center for Health Delivery Innovation, Nemours Children's Health System, Jacksonville, FL, USA

Emmanuel Opati, MBA, MHA, PMP XpertCare Inc., Baltimore, MD, USA

Carlos Pargas, MD Department of Orthopaedics, Nemours/A.I. duPont Hospital for Children, Wilmington, DE, USA

Rameez Qudsi, MD, MPH Department of Orthopaedics, Nemours/A.I. duPont Hospital for Children, Wilmington, DE, USA

Michael Read, MD Candidate UCF College of Medicine '20, Orlando, FL, USA

Suken A. Shah, MD Department of Orthopedic Surgery, Nemours/Alfred I. duPont Hospital for Children, Wilmington, DE, USA

M. Wade Shrader, MD Department of Orthopedic Surgery, Nemours A.I. duPont Hospital for Children, Wilmington, DE, USA

Patricia Solo-Josephson, MD Nemours Children's Health System, Center for Health Delivery Innovation, Orlando, FL, USA

Sean Tackett, MD, MPH Johns Hopkins Bayview Medical Center, Baltimore, MD, USA

Nathan Trexler, ESQ Balick & Balick LLC, Wilmington, DE, USA

Susan Voltz, BS, MBA Nemours Children's Health System, Jacksonville, FL, USA

Cynthia M. Zettler-Greeley, PhD Nemours Children's Health System, Center for Health Delivery Innovation, Orlando, FL, USA

Section I

Basics of Telemedicine

History and Evolution of Telemedicine

John F. Lovejoy III and Michael Read

History of Telemedicine, Evolution of Technology

Origin and Growth of Human Communication

Human communication has constantly evolved with the development of technological advances. Our origins of long-distance communication stem from the basics of fire signals and semaphore (flag waving) and can be traced back to the ancient Greek tragedies or tribal societies [1, 2]. Though the method and function of human communication have changed significantly, there has always been an underlying theme of "patient care." Ancient settlements were known to establish lines of communication in order to bring members of their village into contact with a "physician" stationed in neighboring areas [1].

J. F. Lovejoy III (✉)
Department of Orthopaedics, Sports Medicine and Physical Medicine and Rehabilitation, University of Central Florida School of Medicine, Nemours Children's Hospital, Orlando, FL, USA
e-mail: John.Lovejoy@nemours.org

M. Read
UCF College of Medicine '20, Orlando, FL, USA
e-mail: MRead@knights.ucf.edu

© Springer Nature Switzerland AG 2021　　　　　　3
A. Atanda Jr., J. F. Lovejoy III (eds.), *Telemedicine in Orthopedic Surgery and Sports Medicine*,
https://doi.org/10.1007/978-3-030-53879-8_1

As technology improved, devices were created that allowed for the transmission of information over much larger distances. Three great inventions created the building blocks of modern telemedicine. The first was the telegraph created in the early half of the 1800s [3] by Samuel Morse who assisted in its creation then developed the famous code which bears his name. For the first time, cross-country and transatlantic communication was available in a near instantaneous fashion. During the civil war, these telegraphs were used to transmit casualty lists and to request medical supplies [2]. It is postulated that there were traces of telemedicine at this time, as telegraphs may have been used for medical consults [2].

The next great invention came in 1876 when Alexander Graham Bell patented the first telephone [2]. Shortly afterward, infrastructure was established to allow greater connectivity through phone lines [2]. As telephone technology improved, the ability for individuals to communicate with each other grew exponentially. By 1915, transcontinental telephone service was established [4], and it was not long before telephone lines spread across the country – making coast-to-coast communication possible.

The last part of the trifecta came with the invention of the modern electric television. Invented in 1927 by Philo Taylor Farnsworth, the television added visual communication with sound and allowed real-time broadcasting [5]. By the 1960s, television was being used for closed circuit medical consultations, and telediagnostic clinics were being started [1, 2].

The Birth of Telemedicine

Though there is not a consensus on the true "origin" of telemedicine, there are reports dating back to 1905 when a Dutch physician named Willem Einthoven was receiving ECG readings over long distances [1, 6]. Practices like this continued to grow in popularity across the globe, particularly well documented in France from 1920 to 1940 where radios were used to place medical consults for patients on ships at sea [1, 6]. In the early 1950s, physicians in the United States followed suit by transmitting radiographs to colleagues across the country for evaluation [1]. A notable example is the use of telephone lines to transmit images across 24 miles in eastern Pennsylvania in 1959 [2]. Similar efforts arose and were successful in Canada around the same time, particularly with the well-documented case of radiology consultations of images sent via coaxial cable [2].

The Telemedicine Expansion

Secondary to the success of these early efforts, organized telemedicine began to take hold. In the 1960s, closed circuit television was used for psychiatric consultations between the Nebraska Psychiatric Institute and the Norfolk State Hospital (112 miles apart) [2]. The use of telemedicine continued to expand, with programs now including the radiotelemetry for cardiac monitoring of EKG rhythms [2]. Offshore of the United States, radiographs and EKGs were being sent from ships back to the mainland, eventually expanding to transoceanic transmission [2]. This initial surge of telemedicine was most utilized in rural or underserved communities as a means of providing local physicians with access to specialists unavailable in their area.

Telemedicine soon began to flourish in more urban settings. An early example was the establishment of phone lines by Massachusetts General Hospital which were used to communicate with emergency stations in Logan Airport in the early 1960s [2]. Other programs continued to develop as demonstrated by using phone lines for EKG transmission from the Miami-Dade Fire Department to the University of Miami's Jackson Memorial Hospital starting in 1968 [2].

As technology continued to expand, so too did the accessibility and usefulness of telemedicine. The rise of the Internet in the 1990s established an infrastructure capable of handling large amounts of data in a short period of time [7, 8]. Interestingly, the Internet boom was not associated with an increase in telemedicine efforts. In fact, studies have shown that only one formal telemedicine program that began before 1986 was able to survive into the mid-1990s [2]. In more recent years, there has been a renewed energy behind telemedicine, driven in part by even greater technological expansion as well as an increased demand for specialty physicians in remote areas.

The role of legislation in regulating the medical field has intensified during the twenty-first century. The American Recovery and Reinvestment Act (most specifically a part of it known as the HITECH Act) was signed into law by President Obama in 2009 and began to change the landscape of American medicine almost immediately [9]. The bill promoted the expansion of technology in medicine – particularly through the adoption of electronic medical records (EMRs). It also provided financial incentives to providers who demonstrated "meaningful use" of EMRs [9]. Overall, this legislation was effective in bringing technology into medicine and laid the groundwork for telemedicine to advance into the twenty-first century.

Legislative efforts continued to improve healthcare access through creating "Accountable Care Organizations" with the passage of the Affordable Care Act in 2010. These organizations were tasked with the management of quality of healthcare for Medicare beneficiaries – in which telemedicine and remote monitoring were able to play a substantial role [9]. By 2014, the National Defense Authorization Act was brought into effect. In large part, it focused on telemedicine services specifically geared toward providing care to veterans and helping them to reacclimate. These services have been considered successes, with studies demonstrating that virtual health encounters yield both patient and provider satisfaction rates greater than 90%, along with lowering costs [10].

The growth of telemedicine has accelerated during the last decade, in large part thanks to technological advancements and a renewed energy on gathering funding and creating infrastructure to support telemedicine. As the capability to perform telemedicine increases, it challanges the medical profession to determine how telemedicine fits into today's changing healthcare landscape and to identify what benefits or drawbacks new programs will create.

Advantages and Disadvantages of Telemedicine

Telemedicine presents a unique opportunity to address many of the challenges faced by both providers and patients. Studies demonstrate that 74% of patients would prefer easy access to providers in favor of face-to-face meetings, emphasizing how important convenience has become to the average healthcare consumer [11]. The financial benefits of telemedicine have been well detailed, with studies of individual programs detailing an 11% decrease in clinic costs fueled by less no-shows, attracting new patients, and reducing overhead for operating a practice [11].

One of the most important uses of telemedicine continues to be providing specialty care to underserved and rural communities. Research has shown that for every 100,000 patients in a rural area, there are only 43 specialists available to them [11]. These patients often travel longer distances and are faced with longer wait times while struggling to make appointments. This increased availability involves the patients more in their medical care, leading to fewer missed appointments and better follow-up. Studies have found a measurable benefit of care quality with telemedicine programs. These patients have lower scores on depression, anxiety, and stress scales while having 38% fewer hospital admissions [11].

Telemedicine does come with its own challenges and difficulties. Establishing the infrastructure necessary for telemedicine programs involves extensive training of IT personnel as well as healthcare providers (training initiatives range from $200 to $2000 depending on the complexity of equipment used) [11]. Purchasing equipment is a costly and time-consuming process, with all-in-one systems reaching upward of $28,000 [11].

Additionally, the increase of on-demand healthcare services limits continuity of care. It is always not feasible for each patient to constantly have access to the same provider, which may lead to issues finding previous care notes and establishing strong doctor-patient relationships. This highlights the importance of developing a strong and secure method of accessing patient records across different providers – something that has yet to be developed or implemented at a large scale. Telemedicine consultations may struggle with technical difficulties such as a weak internet connection, leading to communication errors and patient mismanagement. There are also many situations where a physical exam is necessary during a patient encounter, which frequently is not possible over video chat.

Telemedicine has a broad variety of uses and is particularly helpful in situations that do not require in-person communication. As experience with telemedicine solutions increases, the barriers to the setup and maintenance of these programs will become more manageable. Moving toward the next decade, technology has become much less of a barrier to telemedicine – but what is the current trajectory of telemedicine, and how will it fit in to patient care moving forward?

A Changing Healthcare Climate

Researchers and physicians both agree America's growing and aging population will present unique challenges to the US healthcare system. The Centers for Medicare and Medicaid Services (CMS) published a report projecting US healthcare expenditures to increase by 5.5% per year through 2027, eventually reaching a total of $6.0 trillion annually [12]. Furthermore, spending by physician and clinical services is expected to accelerate and grow by 5.4% per year, again fueled by an increased demand for physician services [12].

These statistics offer a glimpse into the need for creative solutions to address the challenges faced by providers and the healthcare system itself. Aside from a strong continuous growth of healthcare utilization, the US healthcare system faces many possible changes in the coming decade. Presidential candidates have placed a large focus on healthcare reform, leaving many questions about the direction of our healthcare system unanswered. The role of telemedicine in the face of changing legislation is difficult to predict; however, trends point toward it being a fundamental part of patient care moving forward.

As detailed previously, telemedicine efforts have been largely successful on a small scale, and many are hopeful that those successes will continue as telemedicine programs expand. In 2019, telemedicine was a $41.4 billion industry which projected to grow by 15.1% annually through 2027 [13]. Initial concerns surrounding telemedicine viewed initial efforts of implementation as a "fad," but the rapid growth of the field suggests it is here to stay. Many of the issues that could plague telemedicine are being addressed, allowing it to adapt to the modern healthcare environment. Concerns surrounding provider reimbursement have been largely quelled, with 32 US states passing laws that allow physicians to be paid similar amounts for telemedicine versus in-person office visits. As greater security solutions continue to develop, patient privacy and HIPAA standards are being met without much difficulty through device encryption and regular security evaluations for health record programs.

While our healthcare system continues to evolve, the role of telemedicine will become clearer. Currently, telemedicine presents itself as a unique opportunity to extend both primary and specialty care to those in hard-to-reach areas. The use of large cloud-based platforms for patient data storage lends itself to greater data analysis for research and easier accessibility to patient records for both providers and the patients themselves. By and large, physicians have already begun to utilize technology in their practices, with over 80% of providers reporting the use of smartphones and medical apps.

Technology has been evolving at a remarkable pace. The widespread availability of smartphones has made face-to-face conversations over long distances accessible to most Americans; however, the prevalence of informal video conferencing raises some ethical questions about defining telemedicine. Although the technology exists in our pockets, how should we define and regulate telemedicine as programs become more commonplace? We argue that formal telemedicine efforts will require a regulatory body that provides certification, guaranteed privacy protection and patient security, and a pool of qualified healthcare providers. Technology will play a large role in the next decade of American healthcare, and it appears that telemedicine will fit well with the changing healthcare landscape.

References

1. Ryu S. History of telemedicine: evolution C, and transformation. Healthc Inform Res. 2010;16(1):65–6. https://doi.org/10.4258/hir.2010.16.1.65.
2. Institute of Medicine (US) Committee on evaluating clinical applications of telemedicine; Field MJ eTAGtATiHCWDNA.
3. Congress Lo. Samuel F. B. Morse papers at the Library of Congress, 1793 to 1919.
4. ScienCentral I, and The American Institute of Physics. A transcontinental telephone line 1999; https://www.pbs.org/transistor/background1/events/transcon.html
5. Stephens M. History of television. https://www.nyu.edu/classes/stephens/History%20of%20Television%20page.htm
6. 2012 Nov 20. 3, The evolution of telehealth: where have we been and where are we going? Available from: https://www.ncbi.nlm.nih.gov/books/NBK207141/BoHCSIoMTRoTiaEHCEWSWDNAPU
7. Rupp S. A quick look at the history of telemedicine. 2017; https://www.nuemd.com/news/2017/01/04/quick-look-history-telemedicine
8. Partners EH. ARRA, The HITECH Act, and meaningful use- an overview. http://excitehealthpartners.com/news/arra-the-hitech-act-and-meaningful-use-an-overview/
9. Waibel KH, Cain SM, Huml-VanZile M, et al. Section 718 (Telemedicine): virtual health outcomes from regional health command Europe. Mil Med. 2019;184(Suppl 1):48–56.
10. eVisit. 10 Pros and cons of telemedicine. 2018.; https://evisit.com/resources/10-pros-and-cons-of-telemedicine/
11. Services CfMaM. National health expenditure data. 2019.
12. Informatics UoTSoB. What are the latest trends in telemedicine in 2018? 2018.
13. Research G. Telemedicine Market Size, Share & Trends Analysis Report By Component, By Delivery Model, By Technology, By Application (Teleradiology, Telepsychiatry), By Type, By End Use, By Region, And Segment Forecasts, 2020 - 20272020.

Telemedicine Regulation and Licensing

2

Carey Officer and Susan Voltz

Introduction

For most of the history of medicine, doctors traveled to their patients. Up through the middle of the last century, physicians "made rounds" by traveling from home to home or from farm to farm.

The tidal change came with the invention of the x-ray machine, something too heavy to put in the back of a horse and buggy or even a car. Large hospitals with sterile operating rooms and specialized nursing skills started popping up in big cities, such as the Johns Hopkins Hospital in Baltimore in 1889. Subsequently, specialists began centering their practices in hospitals or multispecialty clinics, and the patients started traveling to the doctor.

Often, the distances were too great for the ideal doctor-patient relationship, especially for postoperative visits. Harvey Cushing's

C. Officer (✉)
Center for Health Delivery Innovation, Nemours Children's Health System, Jacksonville, FL, USA
e-mail: Carey.Officer@nemours.org

S. Voltz
Nemours Children's Health System, Jacksonville, FL, USA
e-mail: Susan.Voltz@nemours.org

papers from his practice of neurosurgery in Baltimore and Boston circa 1900–1930 are replete with letters exchanged with patients from somewhere in New England or the mid-Atlantic states. Then, 50 years ago, doctors debated whether they should charge for telephone consultations with their patients.

Today, digitalized radiographic images, the electronic medical record, and videoconferencing via Wi-Fi and cellular connections have changed the tide again. With the widespread availability of this enhanced technology, the patient, as well as the doctor, can stay where he/she is.

Specialists congregate in urban centers for good reasons. Facilities are expensive, and so is equipment like MRI scans and operating microscopes. Specialized operating room personnel, nursing staff, and other technicians are needed in critical mass numbers not likely to be found in small towns in order to provide efficient, skilled service 24 hours per day, 7 days per week, thereby creating an environment in which the patient has to travel for any services provided by the central healthcare hub, whether a simple follow-up visit with the doctor or a more complicated operation. But now they don't necessarily need to travel for all services provided by healthcare facilities.

After decades of technological promises, limited fits and starts, telemedicine is no longer the dreamy future or a trumped up gimmick. Telemedicine is here, not only for convenience but for the healthcare needs for our patients, and it makes timely, high-quality healthcare more accessible than at any other time in the history of medicine.

Definition

The American Telemedicine Association, or ATA, doesn't like to define telemedicine or *telehealth* as they are now calling it. They've settled on "Technology-enabled health and care management and delivery systems that extend capacity and access." [1]

That's a definition that could encompass everything from a rectal thermometer to MRI-guided virtual reality surgery carried out transcontinentally over a live Internet connection by advanced robotics. The reason the ATA is so vague is that they do not want possibilities introduced by new technology or new applications to be suffocated by a premature constrictive definition. However, we still need a definition that is workable or at least legal. The Florida Legislature has recently revised their statutes regarding telemedicine and gives the following definition:

> Telehealth is defined as the use of synchronous or asynchronous telecommunications technology by a telehealth provider to provide health care services, including, but not limited to, assessment, diagnosis, consultation, treatment, and monitoring of a patient; transfer of medical data; patient and professional health-related education; public health services; and health administration. Telehealth does not include audio-only telephone calls, e-mail messages, or fax transmissions [2].

Still not crystal clear, is it? But it is much more specific. Let's take it apart and look at the pieces.

First, telehealth uses telecommunications technology beyond the ordinary phone call, mail, or fax. That implies the transmission of images or videos or electronic monitoring data.

Second, telehealth is synchronous or asynchronous. Synchronous telecommunication is in real time like a live video-conference with a patient. Asynchronous telecommunication is sending a set of records and/or digitalized images to a telehealth provider who looks at the data and communicates his/her findings at another time. An online eye exam would be an example.

Third, the healthcare services that can be provided by this means are quite broad, and the language is generous in allowing expansion over the enumerated examples. The clear categories are (1) direct patient care, (2) transfer of medical data, (3) patient and professional health-related education, (4) public health services, and (5) health administration.

The ATA provides a broad definition of telemedicine, and the Florida Legislature provides a legal definition, but what about a working definition? Let's look at the most common services currently provided by telemedicine or telehealth.

The telehealth service most of us imagine is a live interactive consultation with a remote physician via *synchronous videocon-*

ferencing. This could involve physician-to-physician consultation, like an emergency room physician consulting a pediatric orthopedist about a child's injury. Or it could involve a nurse practitioner checking on a patient's wound healing via FaceTime or Skype. An orthopedist may be able to check range of motion and functional status of a joint after physical therapy from anywhere there is an Internet connection.

Communication does not necessarily need to be live. A pediatrician in a remote location may send in photos of a child's spinal exam, a video of his or her gait, and copies of relevant images to an expert in scoliosis while that surgeon is in the operating room and wait for a reply. In the telehealth vernacular, this is called *asynchronous or store-and-forward* transmission.

Another service commonly provided by telehealth is *remote patient monitoring* (RPM). This has been used to monitor blood pressure in hypertensive patients [3] and glucose [4] in diabetic patients who have difficulty getting specialist care due to either distance or physical disability. In orthopedics, sometimes all that is needed is an x-ray to confirm that a fracture or a fusion is healing at the expected time. This can be done at a remote diagnostic testing facility (RDTF), the images are forwarded, and the opinion is relayed back to the patient without the need for transport. Imagine the convenience of this in a spinal cord-injured patient transferred to a rehab hospital after fusion surgery. Not only is the patient spared the time, expense, and discomfort of the transfer, but they also don't lose a day of rehab.

Mobile health or mHealth refers to the use of the Internet and wireless devices to obtain specialized health information. Certainly, anyone can look up anything on WebMD or Wikipedia or get any variety of good and wretchedly bad advice by Googling. But with *mHealth* programs, the patient's doctor can control the flow of accurate information that is specific to the individual patient. Another potential use of *mHealth* programs is online or videoconference peer-to-peer support groups. Sometimes that teenage girl with scoliosis in Hawthorne, Florida, likes to know that she is not alone; there's someone just like her with the same problem in Grand Marais, Minnesota. They should talk. They can talk, if someone takes the time and effort to set up an mHealth program.

Regulation

Medicare and Medicaid

CMS and Medicare guidelines can be accessed on the Internet through the links provided in Appendix A. This is a brief summary of their guidelines.

Medicare pays for specific (Part B) physician or practitioner services furnished through a telecommunications system. Telehealth services substitute for an in-person encounter [5]. This is the good news.

The bad news is that Medicare envisioned telehealth services as a partial solution to limited availability of care in rural areas, so their regulations reflect this.

The most obvious difference between Medicare rules and those of states or private insurance companies is the requirement that the beneficiary be at an approved *originating site* for services to be approved. The originating site must be in a county outside a metropolitan statistical area (MSA) or in a health professional shortage area (HPSA). The CMS provides a website to determine whether the originating site qualifies [6].

There is a special exception as of July 1, 2019, that allows for the individual's home to be an approved originating site for the treatment of substance abuse disorder or a co-occurring mental health disorder. This exception comes with the SUPPORT Act that modifies the Ryan Haight Act governing prescriptions of controlled substances. We can only hope that some future wisdom in Congress will extend the same convenience to patients without addictions.

Another geographic exception as of January 1, 2019, is treatment of acute stroke [7].

Medicare guidelines also specify the type of facility to be an approved originating site. These are hospitals, clinics, dialysis centers, skilled nursing facilities, or community health centers. Homes can be originating sites only for substance abuse disorder, as noted above, or for end-stage renal disease (ESRD) beneficiaries.

Medicare specifies eligible practitioners as doctors, nurse practitioners, physician assistants, nurse-midwives, certified nurse anesthetists, and registered dietitians. Clinical psychologists and clinical social workers also have eligibility to charge for certain services.

Medicare guidelines also specify that eligible telehealth services are provided by live, real-time telecommunications – synchronous services only. Asynchronous services are not covered.

Medicaid guidelines state that telemedicine is viewed as a cost-effective alternative to the more traditional face-to-face way of providing medical care that states can choose to cover under Medicaid. This definition is modeled under Medicare's definition of "telehealth" services. Although the Medicaid statute does not recognize telemedicine as a distinct service, it gives the states wide latitude to cover telehealth services in state applications for Medicaid grants.

State Regulation

Every state has different statutes governing telemedicine, and the legislatures of those states have the option of changing the laws each year, so it is impossible to give specific guidance in each locale. Appendix B contains a link to the Federation of State Medical Boards that contains links to a state-by-state guide to the statutes. It is highly recommended that any new venture in telemedicine consult a law firm with expertise in healthcare before proceeding with their program.

Though every state is different, there are four critical issues that are common to each regulatory agency regarding telemedicine: (1) physician-patient encounter, (2) telepresenter, (3) informed consent, and (4) licensure.

Physician-Patient Encounter

This is telemedicine's most radical departure from traditional medical practice. The doctor-patient relationship is the core value of medicine and has been since ancient times. It involves a face-to-face encounter and physical examination before a diagnosis, treatment, or prognosis can be entertained. This value is codified in most, if not all, medical practice acts. For a viable telemedicine service to exist in any state, an exception must be made to this rule.

The common statutory change is to define telehealth services and then allow a licensed practitioner to use audiovisual technology in a distant location to evaluate, diagnose, and treat patients without the need for a person-to-person encounter or a physical examination. Variations are whether or not another licensed practitioner examines the patient and a full medical history is required or if the patient must make a physical visit to the telehealth provider before or after the telemedicine encounter. Arkansas, for example, requires a pre-existing doctor-patient relationship before the telemedicine encounter, although that relationship can be made through consulting or cross-covering physicians. Texas and Georgia both require an in-person follow-up within a year after a telemedicine encounter.

Telepresenter

The second issue is the presence of a "telepresenter." A telepresenter is a healthcare professional who is with the patient or on the premises during a telemedicine encounter with a remote provider. This is common for cases involving minors but has been removed from most statutes for adults. Texas remains the exception, requiring a healthcare provider to be on the premises but not physically present with the patient during a telemedicine encounter.

Informed Consent

The third issue is informed consent. Twenty states and the District of Columbia require some type of informed consent for telemedicine services. Texas and Washington state require a written, signed consent form.

License Requirements

The fourth issue is licensure requirements. State licenses allow the provider to practice only within state boundaries. Communities that exist on the borders of states have for decades dealt with the confusion that comes from licensing in each individual state. Many practitioners in border towns have simply maintained two licenses. Now telemedicine changes the landscape entirely. The practice of medicine is no longer local with interstate telemedicine encounters becoming more and more common. Telemedicine specialist practitioners usually cannot have a single state license and still provide optimal and efficient care. However, the bureaucratic burden of applying for multiple state licenses can be quite overwhelming.

Recognizing this problem, individual boards and the Federation of State Medical Boards (FSMB) have expanded license options to meet the increasing need for interstate practice. This takes three distinct forms.

First, the District of Columbia, Maryland, New York, Pennsylvania, and Virginia have reciprocity agreements. Any physician licensed in a state that borders on the state that issues the license can practice in that state. So a telemedicine provider in New York could provide services in Connecticut, but a Connecticut provider could not provide services in New York. Furthermore, the Pennsylvania and New York statutes have language that allows this reciprocity exception to apply only to physicians practicing close to the border. Such agreements are helpful only in limited areas.

A more common approach is the use of a conditional or telemedicine license for out-of-state physicians. The licensing state requires the out-of-state provider to be licensed in another state and then obtain a special license to practice telemedicine on residents of the licensing state. A variation on this is the approach taken by Florida, Maine, and New Mexico that requires the out-of-state provider to have a valid license in another state and register as a telemedicine provider.

It should be noted that the specific requirements of each state vary with such things as board certification, history of disciplinary actions, scope of practice, and agreement to follow all applicable statutes in the state issuing the special license or telemedicine registration. For example, Florida allows the practice of telemedicine for an out-of-state licensed provider without registration if (1) in response to an emergent medical condition or (2) in consultation with a

Florida-licensed provider who takes ultimate responsibility for the patient's care.

A more comprehensive solution is multi-state licensure compacts. This solves the problem of telemedicine as well as the more general problem of license portability. The Federation of State Medical Boards (FSMB) assisted in creating the Interstate Medical Licensure Compact (IMLC) in 2013–2014. Twenty-nine states are now participating members, and legislation has been introduced in several more states for future adoption or implementation. The requirements are that (1) an applicant must hold a full, unrestricted medical license in a compact state to serve as the state of principle license (SPL), (2) primary residence is in the SPL state, (3) at least 25% of practice occurs in the SPL state, (4) employer is located in the SPL state, or (5) the SPL is used as residence for US federal income tax purposes [8].

The IMLC provides the most uniform requirements with the widest applications for telemedicine encounters within the member states. Similar compacts have begun for nursing (Enhanced Nursing Licensure Compact by the National Council of State Boards of Nursing) [9], physical therapy (Physical Therapy Licensure Compact by the American Physical Therapy Association) [10], and psychology (Psychology Interjurisdictional Compact by the Association of State and Provincial Psychology Boards) [11]. The legislative trend appears to be gaining momentum, and hopefully the future will provide a more simple landscape for interstate telemedicine.

A special national license for the practice of medicine has been proposed by some policy makers. For a thoughtful discussion of this topic, read "Liberating Telemedicine: Options to Eliminate the State-Licensing Roadblock" by Shirley V. Svorny, PhD [12].

Telehealth Prescribing

All of the above issues involve the regulatory hurdles to the legitimate establishment of the provider-patient relationship and diagnosis via telemedicine services. What about treatment?

There are no barriers to advice and education. Referrals to other providers or treatment programs near the patient can be made without additional regulatory considerations. Possibly physical therapy or psychology treatments by remote providers could be made in specific locales. That leaves surgery and prescriptions.

Current technology does not practically allow for remote surgery, so currently this is not a telemedicine issue.

Prescriptions are not so simple. Each state has guidelines allowing or restricting Internet or interstate prescribing practices. In most states, the process is simply that the prescription must be filled in a pharmacy licensed in the state in which the patient resides, providing a physician-patient relationship has been established. There are two exceptions to this.

One is medications used to induce abortion. At least 19 states ban the use of telemedicine to prescribe such drugs.

More applicable to the practice of orthopedics is the prescription of controlled substances, especially opiate analgesics. Since 2008, the Haight Act, named after an 18-year-old who died of an overdose of prescription painkillers obtained online, has essentially prohibited Internet prescription of controlled substances without a face-to-face encounter. Although the law instructed the DEA to make exception rules for certain specified circumstances, no time constraint accompanied the legislation, and such circumstances were never defined [13]. In response, the medical community trying to treat patients with opioid use disorder (OUD) lobbied for the SUPPORT Act, which was passed this year. SUPPORT requires the attorney general to issue guidelines by October 24, 2019, for "Special Registration" regulations allowing certain providers to use Internet prescribing for treatment of OUD and related mental health conditions [14].

Though regulation of prescribing practices is left to individual states, the language of the federal law dictates that if there is any conflict with the state law, federal law will preempt the state regulation. In other words, the federal law allows Internet prescriptions, so the state law would have to allow for the same, but the provider must meet *at least* the minimum requirements of the federal applicable law.

In general, most states prohibit controlled substance prescriptions based on the patient's completion of an online questionnaire or by telephone and authorize online prescriptions only *if a valid physician-patient relationship has been formed.* Some states list the elements of a valid physician-patient relationship. Other states require the provider to obtain a special authorization before prescribing controlled substances over the Internet. Many states have conditional restrictions, such as whether or not the prescription is intended for chronic or acute pain [15].

Reimbursement

Medicare covers certain encounters as noted above with specific codes and may expand to cover others under the SUPPORT Act [16], such as home treatment for OUD. Many insurance companies cover telehealth encounters in certain circumstances, and some are quite creative.

For example, the Carolinas HealthCare System built a $12 million virtual care center in 2013 to remotely monitor and treat patients across the system's ten ICUs [17]. The center is staffed by intensivists and nurses and has reportedly helped reduce mortality rates by 5% and length of stay by 6%, as well as prevent unnecessary transfers to the CHS hub hospital [18].

At least 32 states require insurance companies to provide reimbursement for telemedicine encounters at the same rate as it does for face-to-face encounters [19]. This is called a "full parity law." A subtle but critical difference is "partial parity." Under partial parity, a private insurer must cover an encounter "on the same basis" as when the service is provided in person.

On the surface, it seems that parity laws encourage the use of telemedicine technology. Insurance companies are forced to cover services that they could have argued were not included in their contracts. However, whenever laws are passed in a field where new technology changes the possibilities dramatically every year, the regulations lag behind and may actually inhibit innovation.

For example, Medicare and 32 states define parity as live videoconferences. But only 23 states (and not Medicare) define asynchronous "store-and-forward" services as telehealth, and only 18 define remote patient monitoring (RPM) as telehealth. Already the national picture is confused as to what services are required to be covered in which states.

Other variations in state law include wording like "terms and conditions" for covered telemedicine services, which allow the insurance companies a great deal of latitude. Partial parity laws, in which the insurer is required to cover a telemedicine service "on the same basis" as a service provided in person, do not allow for coverage of totally new service lines like RPM [20].

A weakness of the parity laws is the codification of the state's definition of telemedicine in a form that restricts future applications. For example, Tennessee requires telemedicine to pay for services only if delivered at "qualified site" such as hospitals, medical offices, federally qualified health clinics, and notably not the home [21]. Kentucky has a telemedicine parity law, but payers are required only to cover services performed by providers affiliated with the telehealth network [22]. Outside that network, the insurers have full discretion on whether or not to cover.

Nineteen states do not have parity laws. This does not mean that telemedicine practices are not thriving in those states. The Carolina Health System virtual ICU was developed in a state without parity laws. The Alabama Stroke Care Network [23], Florida's MDLive program in partnership with Cigna [24], and the Medical University of South Carolina Center for Telehealth Excellence [25] are three examples. In all three, the stakeholders – patients, providers, insurers, and public health agencies – have demonstrated that intelligent innovation and application of telemedicine technology are cost-effective without the hindrance of well-meaning parity law regulation [26].

In summary, telemedicine services are reimbursed in a patchwork fashion reflecting many other facets of medical care in America. The provider needs to be aware of the state regulations in the locale that the patient is located, but there is a reason to believe that cost-effective measures that improve care in the telemedicine arena will win fair reimbursement in the long run.

Privacy

Patients treated under telemedicine encounters have the same right to privacy as patients treated in person. No statutory exceptions have been made. But telemedicine offers new challenges.

Under most traditional care scenarios, doctors, nurses, other professional providers, and the employees of hospitals and clinics are the only ones exposed to private health information (PHI). Through a professional heritage and reinforced by HIPAA regulations, a culture of discretion exists in most care situations in America.

Telemedicine introduces two new variables to privacy concerns. One is the technology itself, and the other is the involvement of others who are not healthcare professionals or employed by healthcare providers. To expand and clarify HIPAA rules, the Health Information Technology for Economic Clinical Health (HITECH) Act of 2009 was passed.

The "covered entities" that must comply to HIPAA requirements are (1) health plans, (2) healthcare providers, (3) healthcare clearing houses, and (4) business associates, such as people or companies contracted to maintain and store medical records, provide legal and accounting services to providers, provide data transmission services for PHI on a routine basis, or otherwise operate as a subcontractor.

As a covered entity, a telemedicine provider is responsible for the security of the technology used to provide the service [27]. This means, as a minimum, security features on software used for telemedicine services and secure wireless networks [28]. But that may not be enough. The burden rests on the covered entity to provide security to PHI. Consultation with an information technology (IT) specialist would be imperative.

The next concern is the expanded use and definition of "business associate." That IT guy you just hired to make sure your system is HIPAA compliant must enter into a business associate agreement (BAA) that ensures his compliance to PHI security.

A grayer area is a "conduit." Skype and You Tube, for example, through their web conferencing applications, have been platforms used to provide telehealth services. So far, those companies have refused to become business associates and define themselves as conduits to transmit information, considering themselves no different than the postal service or the telephone company [29]. The HITECH Act narrowly defines conduit as an entity that transmits information but does not access it except infrequently as necessary to continue to provide the service. This has worked so far, but the potential problem is that the "covered entity," i.e., the telemedicine provider, is required to review records of information system activity and security of tracking systems [30]. In other words, the provider has technical responsibility for the information the "conduit" conducts. Even if a breach never occurs, a covered entity would fail a HIPAA audit and thereby jeopardize reimbursement and continued participation in Medicare/Medicaid programs.

One solution is Microsoft who will offer a BAA to users of the HIPAA-compliant Skype for Business video service. The problem is that each patient, or service site, must have an Office 365 account linked to the Skype for Business account, and the cost is up to $35 per month per user.

A better solution seems to be a secure messaging service (SMS). The apps are likely to be familiar to both the provider and the patient. The log-in system limits access to authorized personnel, and the information transmitted across the system is encrypted. Activity on the network is monitored by a cloud-based platform, thereby fulfilling HIPAA requirements for monitoring information flow and integrity of security [31]. This is inexpensive, easy to use, and HIPAA compliant and currently looks like the technology of the future for telemedicine.

See Appendix C for additional resources.

Liability

Telemedicine is still medicine, and the same responsibilities and the same liability risks still apply. One should stay within their area of expertise, obtain timely consultations, listen carefully, and speak gently. These are the things that always lower risk and improve care. One member of an advisory board at a medical liability company believes that telemedicine risks are low, perhaps even lower than in traditional practice [32]. He believes that the low-risk type encounters (usually telemedicine follow-up office visits as compared to face-to-face ER neural trauma), the paucity of similar prior claims, and the benefits of documentation outweigh any new risks.

On the other hand, though there are few legal opinions specific to telemedicine, three issues seem to have already emerged as potential liability risks [33].

The first is doctor-patient relationship. If a patient feels alienated from the provider and has a bad outcome from his/her disease process, the encounter becomes a risk regardless of whether actual malpractice occurred. In the world of telehealth, the need for an empathetic bedside manner is replaced by the need for an empathetic web-based manner.

The second issue is prescribing. Certain actions, such as prescribing over the Internet to a patient known only by a questionnaire sent online, are not allowed. Awareness of Haight Act requirements and prescribing rules *in the state where the patient resides* is a key to avoiding such liability.

The third issue is licensing. As noted above, the licensing landscape across America is a patchwork. One Pennsylvania practitioner maintains licenses in 18 states, an incredible burden, to care for all his/her patients [34]. It may be easy in a busy practice to end up on a telemedicine encounter with a patient who is not located in a state where the provider is licensed. In this instance, a claim could be filed for practicing without a license, and administrative and criminal censure could conceivably follow.

Although the risks seem low if all the procedures regarding licensing are followed, the prudent practitioner should make sure his/her liability carrier makes a specific clause covering telemedicine activities.

Summary

Telemedicine will become more and more widespread as technology advances and opportunities for cost-effective improvements in care are demonstrated. The technology is changing, and the regulatory environment is following in the usual haphazard way of American medicine. An administrator with knowledge of the current regulatory guidelines, a good technology department, and willingness to provide the best care for patients everywhere are the keys to the future.

Appendix A: Links to Medicare and Medicaid Guidelines

Medicare: https://www.cms.gov/Outreach-and-Education/Medicare-Learning-Network-MLN/MLNProducts/downloads/TelehealthSrvcsfctsht.pdf?utm_campaign=2a178f351b-EMAIL_CAMPAIGN_2019_04_19_08_59&utm_term=0_ae00b0e89a-2a178f351b-353229765&utm_content=90024811&utm_medium=social&utm_source=linkedin&hss_channel=lcp-3619444

Medicaid: https://www.medicaid.gov/medicaid/benefits/telemed/index.html

Appendix B: Link to Federation of State Medical Boards and Telemedicine Policies

Board-by-Board Overview
http://www.fsmb.org/siteassets/advocacy/key-issues/telemedicine_policies_by_state.pdf

Appendix C: Privacy Resources

HIPAA Federal Regulation Codes – 45 CFR Parts 160, 162, and 164: www.hhs.gov/ocr/privacy/hipaa/administrative/combined/

National Institute of Standards and Technology: www.nist.gov/healthcare/

Office of the National Coordinator: www.healthit.gov/

US Department of Health and Human Services: www.hhs.gov/ocr/privacy/index.html

References

1. https://www.americantelemed.org/resource/why-telemedicine/
2. Florida statures, Section 456.47, F.S.
3. Fisher NDL, et al. Development of an entirely remote, non-physician led hypertension management program. Clin Cardiol. 2019;42(2):285–91. https://doi.org/10.1002/clc.23141. Epub 2019 Jan 17.
4. Yaron M, et al. A randomized controlled trial comparing a telemedicine therapeutic intervention with routine care in adults with type 1 diabetes mellitus treated by insulin pumps. Acta Diabetol. 2019;56(6):667–73. https://doi.org/10.1007/s00592-019-01300-1. Epub 2019 Feb 19
5. https://www.cms.gov/Outreach-and-Education/Medicare-Learning-Network-MLN/MLNProducts/downloads/TelehealthSrvcsfctsht.pdf?utm_campaign=2a178f351b-EMAIL_CAMPAIGN_2019_04_19_08_59&utm_term=0_ae00b0e89a-2a178f351b-353229765&utm_content=90024811&utm_medium=social&utm_source=linkedin&hss_channel=lcp-3619444
6. https://data.hrsa.gov/tools/medicare/telehealth
7. https://www.cms.gov/Outreach-and-Education/Medicare-Learning-Network-MLN/MLNMattersArticles/Downloads/MM10883.pdf
8. https://imlcc.org
9. https://www.ncsbn.org/compacts.htm
10. http://www.apta.org/StateIssues/PTLC/
11. https://www.asppb.net/page/PSYPACT
12. https://www.cato.org/sites/cato.org/files/pubs/pdf/pa826.pdf
13. 21 U.S.C. § 829(e); DEA, implementation of the Ryan Haight online pharmacy consumer protection act of 2008, 74 FR 15599-15603 (April 6, 2009).
14. Congressional Research Service, the Special Registration for Telemedicine: In Brief, (December 7, 2018)
15. Kim PL, Cristales KJ, Nash N. Telehealth promises and pitfalls: remote prescribing of controlled substances, the SUPPORT act, and remaining risks. 4/24/2019. https://www.haynesboone.com/publications/telehealth-promises-and-pitfalls
16. https://www.cms.gov/Outreach-and-Education/Medicare-Learning-Network-MLN/MLNProducts/downloads/TelehealthSrvcsfctsht.pdf?utm_campaign=2a178f351b-EMAIL_CAMPAIGN_2019_04_19_08_59&utm_term=0_ae00b0e89a-2a178f351b-353229765&utm_content=90024811&utm_medium=social&utm_source=linkedin&hss_channel=lcp-3619444
17. Thomas J. Carolina HealthCare adds virtual component to intensive care. Charlotte Bus J. 2013 May 23.
18. Tomsic M. Staffing an intensive care unit from miles away has advantages. National Public Radio. 2015 May 6.

19. Center for Connected Health Policy. Telehealth private payer laws: impact and issues. Milbank Memorial Fund. 2017 Aug 23. https://www.milbank.org/publications/telehealth-private-payer-laws-impact-issues/

20. Lacktman N. Examining payment parity in telehealth laws. Health Care Law Today. 2015 Aug 13. https://www.healthcarelawtoday.com/2015/08/13/examining-payment-parity-in-telehealth-laws/

21. Tennessee House Bill 1895. 2014. http://www.capitol.tn.gov/Bills/108/Amend/HA0945.pdf

22. Kentucky Telehealth Administrative Regulations. Accessed Sept. 10, 2017. http://www.lrc.ky.gov/statutes/statute.aspx?id=17373

23. Southeast Alabama Medical Center Stroke Care Network Powerpoint Presentation. Alabama Rural Health and TeleHealth Summit. Oct. 17, 2013. https://www.slideshare.net/gatelehealth/se-al-medical-center

24. Bandell B. MDLIVE to hire dozens in Sunrise after partnership with Cigna. South Florida Bus J. 2013 Apr 23. https://www.bizjournals.com/southflorida/ news/2013/04/23/MDLIVE-to-hire-dozens-in-sunrise-after.html

25. South Carolina Hospital Association. Telemedicine improves access to care in SC. https://www.scha.org/news/telemedicine-improves-access-in-sc

26. Restrepo K. The case against telemedicine parity laws. https://www.johnlocke.org/research/telemedicine/

27. U.S.C. § 164.308 Administrative Safeguards.

28. § 164.312(e)(1) Technical Safeguards.

29. Skype Statement, March 2011. www.onlinetherapyinstitute.com/2011/03/videoconferencing-secure-encrypted-hipaa-compliant/

30. § 164.308(a)(1)(ii)(D) Administrative Safeguards.

31. HIPAA Guidelines on Telemedicine. https://www.hipaajournal.com/hipaa-guidelines-on-telemedicine/

32. McCracken G. How does telemedicine affect malpractice insurance? https://blog.evisit.com/telemedicine-affect-malpractice-insurance

33. Ackerman BG. Is the doctor in? Medical malpractice issues in the age of telemedicine. Nat Law Rev. 2019 Ap 17. https://www.natlawreview.com/article/doctor-medical-malpractice-issues-age-telemedicine

34. Pratt M. How to avoid the legal risks of telemedicine. Med Econ. 2019 June 28. https://www.medicaleconomics.com/authors/mary-k-pratt

Telemedicine Billing and Coding

3

Betty A. Hovey

Introduction

Coding and billing of telemedicine is similar to billing and coding for other professional services performed by physicians and other providers. It requires a knowledge of coding guidelines and payor requirements in order to receive proper payment. Like billing and coding for other services, telemedicine service requirements vary from payor to payor. This chapter will focus on telemedicine billing and coding definitions, guidelines, and various payor requirements.

By 2016, approximately 61% of hospitals and healthcare facilities used telemedicine in the United States [1]. The Centers for Medicare and Medicaid Services (CMS) began paying for telemedicine in 2001. Medicare has specific criteria that must be met in order to bill for telemedicine; commercial payors' guidelines will vary. The *Current Procedural Terminology* (CPT) book also has guidance regarding telemedicine. This includes place of service designation, symbols, and an appendix. All of the different guidelines will be explained for clarity and covered in the following pages.

B. A. Hovey (✉)
Compliant Health Care Solutions, Lemont, IL, USA
e-mail: bettyhovey@chcs.consulting

© Springer Nature Switzerland AG 2021
A. Atanda Jr., J. F. Lovejoy III (eds.), *Telemedicine in Orthopedic Surgery and Sports Medicine*,
https://doi.org/10.1007/978-3-030-53879-8_3

Place of Service

A new place of service (POS) code was added to indicate to a payor that the service was a telemedicine service that was effective on January 1, 2017. This POS should be submitted on a CMS 1500 claim form on professional claims to indicate the service is a telemedicine service. The telemedicine POS code is 02, Telemedicine. The POS descriptor reads, "The location where health services and health related services are provided or received, through a telecommunication system." [2] For example, if a Medicare patient was in a rural hospital's emergency department and the physician was in his/her office, instead of reporting POS 23 for Emergency Room-Hospital, or POS 11 for Office, POS 02 for Telemedicine should be used.

Modifiers

Modifiers are two digit codes appended to a CPT service or procedure code to indicate that the service was modified in some way and there is no CPT code that describes this. Some modifiers are informational and some affect payment. According to *Coding with Modifiers*, modifiers can be used, among other things, to [3]:

- Record a service or procedure that has been modified but not changed in its identification or definition
- Explain special circumstances or conditions of patient care
- Indicate repeat or multiple procedures
- Show cause for higher or lower costs while protecting charge history data
- Report assistant surgeon services
- Report a professional component of a procedure or service

CPT created modifier 95, *Synchronous Telemedicine Service Rendered* via *a Real-Time Interactive Audio and Video Telecommunication System*, to append to any service that is performed remotely. Medicare also created two Healthcare Common Procedure Coding System Level II (HCPCSII) modifiers for telehealth, modifier GT, Via *Interactive Audio and Video Telecommunications Systems*, and modifier GQ, Via *Asynchronous Telecommunications System*, to be appended to the appropriate visit type. When CPT created modifier 95 and place of service code 02 to designate telehealth services, this caused some confusion having two modifiers that give the same information. On November 29, 2017, CMS put out a change request (10153, Transmittal 3929) that stated effective January 1, 2018, modifier GT was not required to append to claims performed via telemedicine [4]. They did not eliminate modifier GQ for asynchronous telemedicine visits. Now there are only two modifiers to choose from: 95 and GQ. So, if a real-time remote patient visit is documented and meets the requirements of 99213, it would be reported as 99213-95. If the same visit is performed as a store-and-forward encounter, it would be reported as 99213-GQ.

Telemedicine Code Symbol

The CPT book uses symbols to signify specific designations that are important in the code set. See Table 3.1 for a listing of important CPT symbols.

Any code that has been preceded by the star ★ symbol may be reported as a telemedicine service according to the American Medical Association (AMA). These codes must be submitted with modifier 95. There are more than 30 codes that the CPT book states may be used to report when performed via telemedicine that are not on Medicare's approved list of telemedicine codes. These include 90832-90838, psychotherapy; 90951-90952, 90954-90955, 90957-90958, end stage renal disease services; and 92227–92228, remote imaging and monitoring of retinal disease.

Appendix P

In the official AMA CPT book, there is an appendix that lists all of the codes that have the star symbol in front of them – Appendix P. This appendix allows a practice to see all of the AMA-approved codes for telemedicine in one place. This list does not coincide

Table 3.1 Important CPT symbols

Symbol	Description	Purpose
•	New code	Used when new procedure codes are added to the CPT book
▲	Revised code	Used when a code revision has resulted in a substantial alteration to the CPT descriptor
+	Add-on code	Used to indicate that the CPT code is an add-on code, which cannot be reported alone
⌀	Modifier 51 exempt code	Used to indicate that the code is exempt from appending modifier 51
⚡	FDA approval pending	Used when a CPT code is for a vaccine that is pending FDA approval
#	Resequenced code	Used when a code is not placed numerically in the CPT book
★	Telemedicine services	Used to indicate the code may be reported as a telemedicine service

with Medicare's approved telemedicine codes, so it is imperative with commercial payors to query a payor and find out which codes they cover.

Medicare

The Medicare, Medicaid, and State Children's Health Insurance Program Benefits Improvement and Protection Act of 2000 (BIPA) included an amendment in Section 223 to provide the basis for Medicare's coverage of telemedicine [5]. This drove Medicare in 2001 to pay for remote consultations, office visits, and psychiatry services. All of the different criteria that Medicare has introduced into their guidelines in order to receive payment for telemedicine will be discussed.

Key Definitions

It is important to understand the basic definitions Medicare uses for telemedicine services to ensure that billing of those services is done compliantly. The following are the important definitions one needs to know in order to bill telemedicine correctly [6, 7]:

- *Originating site* – the location of an eligible Medicare beneficiary at the time the service being furnished via a telecommunication system occurs.
- *Distant site* – the site where the physician or practitioner providing the professional services is located at the time the service is provided via a telecommunication system.
- *Synchronous service* – remote service performed using interactive audio and video telecommunication system that permits real-time communication between physician/practitioner and patient.
- *Asynchronous service* – also called "store and forward," a remote service in which documents (records, labs, images, etc.) are collected and transmitted to a physician/practitioner not using synchronous real-time telecommunication which the physician/practitioner reviews and gives feedback. Medicare only pays for asynchronous telemedicine if it is part of a Federal telemedicine demonstration project in the states of Alaska and/or Hawaii.

Site Requirements

Medicare currently does not pay for telemedicine visits when the patient is in their home. In fact, Medicare has very specific site requirements. In order to get paid for a telemedicine office visit or consultation, the patient must be either in a county outside a metropolitan statistical area (MSA) or a rural health professional shortage area (HPSA) in a rural census tract. An MSA is defined by the US Office of Management and Budget (OMB) as one or more adjacent counties or county equivalents that have at least 50,000 population plus adjacent territory that has a high degree of social and economic integration with the core as measured by community ties. OMB recognizes 384 MSAs for the United States and 8 for Puerto Rico [8].

A HPSA is defined by CMS as a geographic area, or populations within a geographic area, that lacks sufficient healthcare providers (primary care, dental, or mental health) to meet the healthcare needs of the area population. A HPSA is designated based on census tracts by the Health Resources and Services Administration (HRSA) [9].

Approved originating sites within these areas are as follows:

1. Physician and practitioner offices
2. Hospitals
3. Critical access hospitals (CAHs)
4. Rural health clinics
5. Federally qualified health centers
6. Hospital-based or CAH-based renal dialysis centers (including satellites)
7. Skilled nursing facilities (SNFs)
8. Community mental health centers (CMHCs)
9. Renal dialysis facilities
10. Homes of beneficiaries with end-stage renal disease (ESRD) getting home dialysis
11. Mobile stroke units

Approved distant site practitioners who can furnish and get paid for covered telehealth services within these areas are as follows:

1. Physicians
2. Nurse practitioners (NPs)
3. Physician assistants (PAs)
4. Nurse-midwives
5. Clinical nurse specialists (CNSs)
6. Certified registered nurse anesthetists (CRNAs)
7. Clinical psychologists (CPs) and clinical social workers (CSWs)
8. Registered dietitians or nutrition professional

Remember, Medicare only pays for real-time communication (synchronous) telemedicine in the approved areas above, unless the practice is involved with an asynchronous (store-and-forward) Federal demonstration project in Alaska or Hawaii.

Covered Services

Medicare pays for specific service performed remotely. A full list of covered services for 2020 can be found at https://www.cms. gov/Medicare/Medicare-General-Information/Telehealth/ Telehealth-Codes. Table 3.2 contains a list of the visits Medicare will pay for when done via telemedicine.

Code Q3014, telehealth originating site facility fee, may be billed to Medicare in addition to any other services the site performs for the patient during the telemedicine encounter. For 2020, the Medicare payment for Q3014 is $26.65.

The Health Resources and Services Administration has a webpage available to check if the originating site is valid for telemedicine coverage [10]. This webpage allows a practice to input the full address of the site the patient will be during the telemedicine encounter, click the Search button, and then a message will display that states the site is, or is not, eligible for Medicare telehealth payment.

Medicare has frequency limits to some telemedicine services. For telemedicine, subsequent hospital care services are limited to one every 3 days, and subsequent nursing facility services are limited to one every 30 days.

In order to bill Medicare for a telemedicine visit, the following criteria must be met:

1. The patient must be an eligible beneficiary.
2. The patient must be in an approved originating site.
3. The distant site practitioner must be an approved type (physician, NP, etc.).
4. The visit must be performed using an interactive telecommunications system (unless in asynchronous Federal demonstration project in Alaska or Hawaii).
5. The patient must give consent for the telemedicine service (can be verbal, but must document it).

Table 3.2 Telemedicine covered visit codes (not an all-inclusive list of covered services)

CPT/HCPCS II Code	Descriptor
99201	Office/outpatient visit new level 1
99202	Office/outpatient visit new level 2
99203	Office/outpatient visit new level 3
99204	Office/outpatient visit new level 4
99205	Office/outpatient visit new level 5
99211	Office/outpatient visit established level 1
99212	Office/outpatient visit established level 2
99213	Office/outpatient visit established level 3
99214	Office/outpatient visit established level 4
99215	Office/outpatient visit established level 5
99231	Subsequent hospital care level 1
99232	Subsequent hospital care level 2
99233	Subsequent hospital care level 3
99307	Nursing fac care subsequent straightforward MDM
99308	Nursing fac care subsequent low MDM
99309	Nursing fac care subsequent moderate MDM
99310	Nursing fac care subsequent high MDM
99354	Prolonged service office first hour
99355	Prolonged service office each additional 30 minutes
99356	Prolonged service inpatient first hour
99357	Prolonged service inpatient each additional 30 minutes
G0406	Inpt/tele follow-up 15 minutes
G0407	Inpt/tele follow-up 25 minutes
G0408	Inpt/tele follow-up 35 minutes
G0425	Inpt/ed teleconsult 30 minutes
G0426	Inpt/ed teleconsult 50 minutes
G0427	Inpt/ed teleconsult 70 minutes
G0438	Annual wellness visit, initial visit
G0439	Annual wellness visit, subsequent visit
G0508	Crit care telehea consult, initial, 60 minutes
G0509	Crit care telehea consult, subsequent, 50 minutes
G0513	Prolong prev svcs, first 30 minutes
G0514	Prolong prev svcs, each additional 30 minutes

6. Documentation must support the level of service reported.
7. The service performed must be on the covered services list for telemedicine.
8. The service is billed with modifier 95 appended to the code(s) reported, and place of service 02 (telemedicine) is submitted.

Commercial Payors

When it comes to telemedicine coverage, commercial payors' guidelines will vary, just as with any other services. Some states have no regulations on coverage for telemedicine services, others have limited coverage, and still others have broad coverage.

According to 50-State Survey of Telehealth Commercial Payer Statutes (2019), 42 states and the District of Columbia currently have telehealth commercial payer statutes [11]. Some of the things to look for in the laws regarding telemedicine are as follows:

1. *Coverage provision* – Some laws have a provision on coverage parity, which means that the payor must cover a healthcare service delivered by means of telemedicine if they would cover it if it were provided as an in-person service.
2. *Reimbursement provision* – Some laws have a reimbursement provision, which states how the commercial insurer must pay for telemedicine services. Some provisions state that a telemedicine service must be paid the same rate as they do for in-person services. Some allow a percentage "discount" for telemedicine services due to lack of overhead. Some laws set a maximum payment, while others set a minimum.
3. *Cost-shifting protection for plan members* – Some laws give cost-shifting protection against a payor charging higher deductible, co-insurance, or co-pays for a telemedicine visit.
4. *Originating site designation* – Some laws may adopt the Medicare originating site designations, while others may expand on it to allow patient's access to telemedicine visits from more locations (patient's home, etc.).

5. *Remote patient monitoring* – Some states' laws include provisions for remote patient monitoring. Some laws require payors to cover things like virtual check-ins, remote monitoring of physiologic parameters, and remote physiologic monitoring and treatment.
6. *Asynchronous telemedicine* – Some laws require payors to cover store-and-forward telemedicine.
7. *Patient type* – Some laws require that a patient receiving a telemedicine service be an established patient to the physician/practitioner providing the service.
8. *Narrow/exclusive/in-network provider limits* – Some laws have language that addresses if a payor may limit coverage and/or reimbursement for telemedicine services to only those practitioners that are within the payor's narrow telehealth network. What this means is that a payor may be allowed to deny payment for telemedicine to out-of-network physicians.

Besides the state laws, each payor may have their own policies regarding telemedicine. For example, Blue Cross Blue Shield has added the patient's residence as an approved originating site in their policy, while UnitedHealthcare only allows the patient's home as an approved site if the patient is having monthly end-stage renal disease (ESRD) and ESRD-related clinical assessments and for treatment of a substance use disorder or a co-occurring mental health disorder [12, 13].

Medicaid

Since Medicaid is subject to state law, the rules for Medicaid will vary state by state, with no two states being alike. According to the Center for Connected Health Policy's Fall 2019 state telehealth laws survey, state Medicaid agencies are addressing telehealth [14]. Highlights of the survey include:

- All 50 states and Washington, DC, offer payment for some form of live video in the Medicaid fee-for-service plans.
- Fourteen states pay for asynchronous (store-and-forward) telemedicine.

- Twenty-two state Medicaid programs pay for remote patient monitoring (RPM).
- Twenty-three states have limitations of what type of facility will be considered as an originating site.

When offering telemedicine, it is important to understand the laws of the state(s) where the practice is located and different payor policies and requirements. The more research and preparation that is done ahead of time, the better it will be for the practice.

Interstate Licensure for Telemedicine

In order to deliver healthcare services to a patient, a physician or other practitioner must have a license in the state where the patient is receiving medical services. The same is true for telemedicine. So, while the technology can allow for interstate treatment via telemedicine for patients, a physician's license does not. Some states, like Maryland and New York, allow licensure reciprocity with bordering states. State boards can also issue special purpose licenses, telemedicine licenses/certificates, or licenses to practice medicine across state lines to provide telemedicine services under certain circumstances. For example, Texas has an out-of-state telemedicine license that specifically limits the license holder to two services:

1. The interpretation of diagnostic testing and reporting the results to a Texas fully licensed physician practicing in Texas
2. The follow-up of patients where the majority of the patient care was rendered in another state

The Interstate Medical Licensure Compact (IMLC) can also assist with getting licensure for physicians wanting to offer telemedicine to patients in other states. The compact was created by the Federation of State Medical Boards and offers a streamlined licensing process for physicians wishing to practice across state lines, including telemedicine services [15]. Currently, 29 states are part of the compact, and more states have introduced compact legislation.

Conclusion

Here are suggested steps to take if your practice wishes to bill for telemedicine services:

1. Contact the state medical board and ask for the state policies on telehealth.
2. Contact the state licensing board, and obtain the rules about Reciprocity Agreements and Interstate Medical Licensure Compacts.
3. Understand the Federal guidelines on telemedicine. Download and review CMS telehealth reimbursement guidelines.
4. Research policies of commercial payors regarding telemedicine. Download any coverage policies for review.
5. Organize the Medicare and commercial data collected into a chart that shows which plans reimburse for telehealth, the documentation and claim filing rules for each, and any coding and billing rules. Having a reference chart of the details will improve staff efficiency and billing accuracy.
6. Develop a patient disclosure statement. It may be helpful to enlist a healthcare attorney. Each patient scheduled for a telehealth visit will need to sign one.

Coding telemedicine services is not difficult; it is coded just as if the patient were present. The billing of telemedicine services is much more involved.

References

1. US Department of Health and Human Services. Report to Congress: e-health and telemedicine. aspe.hhs.gov/system/files/pdf/206751/TelemedicineE-HealthReport.pdf. Accessed 1 Dec 2019.
2. CPT 2020, Professional Edition. 2020. The American Medical Association.
3. Grider D. Coding with modifiers: a guide to correct CPT and HCPCS level II modifier usage: American Medical Association; 2011.

4. Medicare, Medicaid, and SCHIP Benefits Improvement Act of 2000. 2000. https://www.govtrack.us/congress/bills/106/hr5661/text. Accessed 1 Dec 2019.
5. Center for Medicare and Medicaid Services. Medicare claims processing manual chapter 12- Physician/Nonphysician Practitioners. https://www.cms.gov/Regulations-and-Guidance/Guidance/Manuals/Downloads/clm104c12.pdf. Accessed 1 Dec 2019.
6. Medicare Learning Network. 2019. Telehealth Services. https://www.cms.gov/Outreach-and-Education/Medicare-Learning-Network-MLN/MLNProducts/Downloads/TelehealthSrvcsfctsht.pdf. Accessed 1 Dec 2019.
7. United States Government Publishing Office. (2010). Federal register part IV office of management and budget; 2010 Standards for delineating metropolitan and micropolitan statistical areas. https://www.govinfo.gov/content/pkg/FR-2010-06-28/pdf/2010-15605.pdf. Accessed 1 Dec 2019.
8. Health Professional Shortage Area Physician Bonus Program. December, 2017. https://www.cms.gov/Outreach-and-Education/Medicare-Learning-Network-MLN/MLNProducts/downloads/HPSAfctsht.pdf. Accessed 1 Dec 2019.
9. Medicare Telehealth Payment Eligibility Analyzer. 2019. https://data.hrsa.gov/tools/medicare/telehealth. Accessed 1 Dec 2019.
10. Lacktman et al. 50-state survey of telehealth commercial payer statutes; 2019. Retrieved from Foley & Lardner LLC. https://www.foley.com/-/media/files/insights/health-care-law-today/19mc21486-50state-survey-of-telehealth-commercial.pdf. Accessed 1 Dec 2019.
11. Pub 100-04 Medicare Claims Processing Manual. 2017. Retrieved from https://www.cms.gov/Regulations-and-Guidance/Guidance/Transmittals/2017Downloads/R3929CP.pdf. Accessed 1 Dec 2019.
12. Telemedicine Medical Services and Telehealth Services. 2019. Retrieved from Blue Cross Blue Shield of Texas. https://www.bcbstx.com/provider/pdf/txcpcp01_telemedicine_and_telehealth_servces_new.pdf. Accessed 1 Dec 2019.
13. Telehealth and Telemedicine Policy, Professional. 2019. Retrieved from uhcprovider.com. https://www.uhcprovider.com/content/dam/provider/docs/public/policies/comm-reimbursement/COMM-Telehealth-and-Telemedicine-Policy.pdf. Accessed 1 Dec 2019.
14. State Telehealth Laws & Reimbursement Policies Fall 2019. 2019. Retrieved from Center for Connected Health Policy. https://www.cchpca.org/sites/default/files/2019-10/50%20State%20Telehalth%20Laws%20and%20Reibmursement%20Policies%20Report%20Fall%202019%20FINAL.pdf. Accessed 1 Dec 2019.
15. The IMLC. 2019. Retrieved from ilmcc.org. https://imlcc.org/. Accessed 1 Dec 2019.

Legal Compliance in Telemedicine

4

Nathan Trexler

Introduction

The use of telemedicine is rapidly expanding and can offer valuable new ways in which patients and their healthcare providers can manage healthcare needs. Physicians may wish to offer telemedicine within their practices to established patients, or physicians may wish to join any number of rapidly growing networks that offer patients access to specialists where such access may have been historically limited, due to geography, cost, or other factors. Whatever the driving force behind the desire to explore the use of telemedicine, physicians should be keenly aware of the legal barriers or limitations prior to initiating or expanding the use of telemedicine in delivering medical care to patients.

This chapter identifies and discusses several issues for physicians to consider prior to engaging in telemedicine practice, whether it be in establishing a telemedicine program in a practice or facility-based setting or participating in any number of nationwide networks connecting physicians and patients. Primarily, this

N. Trexler (✉)
Balick & Balick LLC, Wilmington, DE, USA
e-mail: ntrexler@balick.com

© Springer Nature Switzerland AG 2021
A. Atanda Jr., J. F. Lovejoy III (eds.), *Telemedicine in Orthopedic Surgery and Sports Medicine*,
https://doi.org/10.1007/978-3-030-53879-8_4

chapter will identify common issues that must be analyzed using Delaware and federal law as a guide. This chapter will address state licensure requirements and practice standards, including forming physician-patient relationships, informed consent, and limitations on the use of telemedicine. Next, the chapter will turn to the implications of federal fraud and abuse laws, including the federal Anti-Kickback Statute and the federal Physician Self-Referral Law, commonly known as the Stark Law.

While physicians should always consider how applicable state law specifically defines certain key terms related to telemedicine, it is useful for this chapter to generally define certain terms for purposes of the following discussion. First, this chapter will generally refer to the location of the patient participating in telemedicine as the originating site and the location of the physician rendering telemedicine services as the distant site.

It is important to note that the law regarding telemedicine is evolving and may, potentially, ease some of the burdens related to multi-state telemedicine practices but may also respond to new concerns related to such practices. Physicians should always consult applicable state licensing boards or legal counsel for up-to-date requirements and permissible practices. This chapter is intended to convey general information only and not to provide legal advice. The information contained herein may not reflect current legal developments and should not be relied upon without consulting legal counsel.

What Law Applies?

Where the physician rendering services through telemedicine is located in a state different than where the patient is physically located, the question often asked by physicians is which state's law will regulate the physician's conduct. Does the law of the state in which the patient is located or the state in which the physician is located apply? States have an interest in regulating the practice of medicine within their jurisdictions, with protection of the public as its overriding interest, and licensure is the primary means of regulation.

For this reason, the location of the patient (or the originating site) will generally determine the state law that will govern the physician's interactions with respect to that patient (or with another physician) even if the physician is located elsewhere (the distant site) in another state. Often times, state law will make this clear. For example, Delaware law defines the practice of medicine to include "rendering a written or otherwise documented medical opinion concerning the diagnosis or treatment of a person or the actual rendering of treatment *to a person within the State by a physician located outside the State* as a result of transmission of the person's medical data by electronic or other means from within the State to the physician or to the physician's agent."[1] Such a definition is designed to make it clear that interstate practice via telemedicine is regulated by Delaware law when the patient is physically located in Delaware regardless of where the physician is located. In other circumstances, a state's law may not be as clear, but the informed position is that the originating site's state law will apply.

Physicians should familiarize themselves with several sources of information within each state regarding the regulation of physicians, generally, and telemedicine, specifically. These include:

1. State medical practice acts (statutes)
2. State insurance statutes (regarding public and commercial coverage and reimbursement requirements)
3. State medical board regulations
4. State medical board websites and formal or informal opinions regarding the practice of medicine and telemedicine, specifically

For physicians that seek to render telemedicine services in multiple states, quite a bit of due diligence will be necessary.

---

[1] 24 Del. Code § 1702(12).

State Licensure

Knowing that the originating site's state law will apply, before rendering telemedicine services, the physician must consider whether he or she will be engaged in the "practice of medicine," generally, or "telemedicine," specifically, as those terms are defined by law and/or regulation in that state and whether or not a license is required. If the physician is not engaged in the practice of medicine (or telemedicine) in the state of the originating site, the analysis essentially ends.

States often define the "practice of medicine" broadly. For example, Delaware defines the "practice of medicine" as including the following:

1. Advertising, holding out to the public, or representing in any manner that one is authorized to practice medicine in this state
2. Offering or undertaking to prescribe, order, give, or administer any drug or medicine for the use of another person
3. Offering or undertaking to prevent or to diagnose, correct, and/or treat in any manner or by any means, methods, or devices a disease, illness, pain, wound, fracture, infirmity, defect, or abnormal physical or mental condition of another person, including the management of pregnancy and parturition
4. Offering or undertaking to perform a surgical operation upon another person
5. Rendering a written or otherwise documented medical opinion concerning the diagnosis or treatment of a person or the actual rendering of treatment to a person within the state by a physician located outside the state as a result of transmission of the person's medical data by electronic or other means from within the state to the physician or to the physician's agent
6. Rendering a determination of medical necessity or a decision affecting or modifying the diagnosis and/or treatment of a person
7. Using the designation doctor, doctor of medicine, doctor of osteopathy, physician, surgeon, physician and surgeon, Dr., M.D., or D.O., or a similar designation, or any combination

thereof, in the conduct of an occupation or profession pertaining to the prevention, diagnosis, or treatment of human disease or condition, unless the designation additionally contains the description of another branch of the healing arts for which one holds a valid license in the state.[2]

Not every state defines the practice of medicine so broadly, but in nearly every circumstance, it will include the diagnosis and treatment of a patient.

"Telemedicine" is usually defined more specifically, as is the case in Delaware, where "telemedicine" means "a form of tele-health which is the delivery of clinical health-care services by means of real time 2-way audio, visual, or other telecommunications or electronic communications, including the application of secure video conferencing or store and forward transfer technology to provide or support health-care delivery, which facilitate the assessment, diagnosis, consultation, treatment, education, care management and self-management of a patient's health care by a health-care provider practicing within his or her scope of practice as would be practiced in-person with a patient, legally allowed to practice in the State, while such patient is at an originating site and the health-care provider is at a distant site."[3]

While it may seem impossible to render services to a patient that will not implicate the practice of medicine, particularly given Delaware's broad definition, technology companies that engage physicians to render services to the companies' customers may seek to limit the nature of the services to avoid the licensure hurdle. In other words, the company may limit the scope of work to avoid the actual practice of medicine, even if using traditional telemedicine technologies and platforms. The best example of this is the educational approach, where such services may seek to be solely informational in nature and not involve, for example, establishing a diagnosis or recommending a particular treatment. Physicians should carefully approach such arrangements and

---

[2] 24 Del. Code § 1702(12).
[3] 24 Del. Code § 1702(17); 18 Del. Code § 3370(a)(5).

consider the precise scope of work to determine whether it will be considered the practice of medicine necessitating licensure.

If the physician engages in telemedicine in the state of the originating site, the physician is generally required to obtain a license from that state. However, there are common exceptions to the licensure requirement. For example, most states have a consultation exception that allows for an unlicensed physician to consult provider to provider with a physician licensed in the originating state. In such cases, it is usually contemplated that the local, licensed physician will retain control of the treatment of the patient. While such an exception is available in most states, the scope of the exception can vary widely, necessitating individualized consideration.

For example, in Delaware, licensing is not required for a physician licensed in another state or foreign country consulting with a physician licensed in Delaware.[4] Compare this exception to, for example, Arizona, where licensing is not required for a "doctor of medicine residing in another jurisdiction who is authorized to practice medicine in that jurisdiction, if the doctor engages in actual single or infrequent consultation with a doctor of medicine licensed in" Arizona if the consultation is with respect to a specific patient or patients.[5] Similarly, in New Hampshire, a physician licensed in another state that is called in consultation by a New Hampshire-licensed physician shall not be required to hold a license as long as such consultation is not "regular or frequent" as determined by the New Hampshire Board of Medicine.[6] Notably, Delaware does not have frequency limitations like Arizona or New Hampshire. Moreover, unlike in Delaware, some states clearly require that the licensed physician must retain ultimate authority over the treatment of the patient. For example, in California, the non-licensed physician, while permitted to consult with a California-licensed physician, may expressly not "have ultimate authority over the care or primary diagnosis of a patient

---

[4] 24 Del. C. § 1727.

[5] Ariz. Rev. Stat. § 32-1421.

[6] N.H. Rev. Stat. Ann. § 329:21.

who is located within" California.[7] Other variations on this provider-to-provider consultation exception include whether the non-licensed physician may be compensated for the consultation and whether there must be a contractual arrangement between the out-of-state consulting physician and the in-state physician.

When it comes to rendering services directly to patients, as opposed to provider-to-provider consults, the licensing requirements are far clearer. If the physician performs services or engages in conduct via telemedicine technology that the state would conclude is the practice of medicine, licensing is required, although some states allow for special, abbreviated licenses or registrations that allow for the practice of telemedicine across state lines. In Delaware, full licensure is required. However, in Minnesota, for example, a physician licensed elsewhere may register with the Minnesota Board of Medical Practice to provide telemedicine services to patients located in Minnesota if:

1. The physician is licensed without restriction to practice medicine in the state from which the physician provides telemedicine services.
2. The physician has not had a license to practice medicine revoked or restricted in any state or jurisdiction.
3. The physician does not open an office in this state, does not meet with patients in this state, and does not receive calls in this state from patients.
4. The physician annually registers with the board, on a form provided by the board.[8]

Given that licensure is often considered a barrier to expansion of telemedicine, physicians should routinely investigate legal developments in each state where they intend to render services by telemedicine. One sign that the licensure burdens are easing is the Interstate Medical Licensure Compact, which offers an expedited pathway to licensure across multiple states. Currently, there

---

[7]Cal. Bus. & Prof. Code § 2060.
[8]Minn. Stat. Ann. § 147.032.

are 24 states accepting applications for multi-state licensure under the compact, making obtaining a medical license in these states more streamlined if a physician already holds a primary license in a participating state. Such developments will ease some of the barriers to engaging in telemedicine across state lines, and this trend is expected to continue.

Scope of Telemedicine and Practice Standards

The next consideration is the scope of telemedicine or, perhaps more pointedly, the limitations on telemedicine practice and the applicable standards as established by the state of the originating site. This includes whether a physician can establish (and if so, how) a patient-physician relationship via telemedicine, informed consent, and limitations on the types of items and services that can be delivered via telemedicine. Again, as with licensure, the originating site's state law will control.

Establishing a Physician-Patient Relationship via Telemedicine

All states require that a physician-patient relationship exist prior to rendering services by telemedicine, although the requirements for forming a physician-patient relationship vary from state to state. Most states do not require an in-person examination to establish the relationship, but there are exceptions to this rule, particularly if the patient's medical condition necessitates an in-person examination. For example, if, during an initial telemedicine encounter, it becomes clear that an in-person examination is necessary to establish the treatment relationship, states, including Delaware, expect the physician to end the encounter and instruct the patient to follow up in person with the physician or another practitioner.

In Delaware, a physician may not utilize telemedicine in the absence of a physician-patient relationship, *except* in the following situations:

1. Informal consultation performed by a physician outside the context of a contractual relationship and on an irregular or infrequent basis without the expectation or exchange of direct or indirect compensation
2. Furnishing of medical assistance by a physician in case of an emergency or disaster if no charge is made for the medical assistance
3. Episodic consultation by a medical specialist located in another jurisdiction who provides such consultation services on request to a licensed healthcare professional[9]

If an exception does not apply, a physician-patient relationship must be established. In Delaware, a physician is not required to establish a physician-patient relationship in person, unless required by the patient's medical condition. The relationship may be formed using live, real-time audio and visual communication or by meeting standards for establishing a relationship as included in evidenced-based clinical practice guidelines in telemedicine developed by major medical specialty societies that are members of the Council of Medical Specialty Societies.[10] Some discretion is given to consider the case-by-case circumstances to determine the requirements for establishing that relationship. "[I]f such action would otherwise be required in the provision of the same service" delivered in person, the physician must establish the relationship either in person or through telemedicine to include (but not necessarily be limited to) the following requirements:

1. Fully verifying and authenticating the location and, to the extent possible, identifying the requesting patient
2. Disclosing and validating the provider's identity and applicable credential or credentials
3. Obtaining appropriate informed consent
4. Establishing a diagnosis through the use of acceptable medical practices, such as patient history, mental status examination,

---

[9]24 Del. Code § 1769D(a) and (k).

[10]24 Del. Code § 1769D(h); 24 Del. Admin. Code §19.4.

physical examination (unless not warranted by the patient's mental condition), and appropriate diagnostic and laboratory testing to establish diagnoses, as well as identify underlying conditions or contraindications, or both, to treatment recommended or provided

5. Discussing with the patient the diagnosis and the evidence for it and the risks and benefits of various treatment options
6. Ensuring the availability of the distant site provider or coverage of the patient for appropriate follow-up care
7. Providing a written visit summary to the patient[11]

Once a physician-patient relationship is established, Delaware law does not require that the physician's subsequent treatment of the same patient satisfy the same requirements.[12]

Other states take similar approaches. For example, in Iowa, physicians may establish a physician-patient relationship "through telemedicine, if the standard of care does not require an in-person encounter, and in accordance with evidence-based standards of practice and telemedicine practice guidelines that address the clinical and technological aspects of telemedicine."[13] In other words, an in-person examination is not required to establish the relationship, unless it is.

Other states are clear about what will *not* suffice to establish a physician-patient relationship. For example, Arkansas law specifically states the following means will not be sufficient to establish a physician-patient relationship: (1) by Internet questionnaire; (2) by email; (3) by patient-generated medical history; (4) by audio-only communication, including, without limitation, interactive audio; (5) by text messaging; (6) by facsimile; or (7) by any combination of these methods.[14]

Physicians should clearly understand the state's legal requirements as well as the evidence-based standards. The policies and

---

[11]24 Del. Code § 1769D(b).

[12]24 Del. Code § 1769D(i).

[13]Iowa Admin. Code § 653-13.11(14).

[14]Ark. Code Ann. § 17-80-403.

procedures, based on these requirements and standards, can be prepared for consistent application in the practice via telemedicine.

Informed Consent

Informed consent is not a new topic for physicians, but informed consent in telemedicine is about obtaining consent for the *manner* in which services are delivered, not necessarily the recommended treatment itself.

Under Delaware law, the physician must obtain a specific consent to utilize telemedicine technologies after disclosures regarding the delivery model and treatment methods and the potential limitations thereof.[15] Some states require that informed consent be in writing (like Colorado), and other states (like Delaware) permit either oral or written informed consent. Practically, the informed consent form should disclose what telemedicine is, who the physician is, what the technology is and how it will be used, and what information may be shared via telemedicine. The benefits of telemedicine and the risks must be disclosed, including what a patient should do in an emergency.

Some states have specific informed consent requirements for Medicaid coverage that may differ from general practice requirements. Physicians should become familiar with the requirements and draft compliant forms to utilize with patients.

Prescribing

Prescribing controlled substances via telemedicine is one of the more common treatments rendered via telemedicine that includes limitations and is one of the few circumstances where federal law, in addition to state law, comes into play.

---

[15] 24 Del. Code § 1769D(b)(3).

In 2008, the Ryan Haight Online Pharmacy Consumer Protection Act (the "Ryan Haight Act") was signed into law. Under the Ryan Haight Act, prescribing of controlled substances via telemedicine is prohibited unless at least one in-person examination is performed or an exception is met. The exceptions relate to the practice of telemedicine conducted in certain practice scenarios. The scenarios include (1) while the patient is physically located in a hospital or clinic and treated by a practitioner acting in accordance with state law and registered in the state in which the patient is located and (2) while the patient is being treated by and in the physical presence of another registered practitioner acting in accordance with state law.

Physicians should carefully review the exceptions to determine whether prescribing a controlled substance without an in-person examination is permissible under federal law. Each of these exceptions is dependent upon compliance with state laws, which are highly variable. In Delaware, a physician may not prescribe an opioid via telemedicine except within an addiction treatment program that received a waiver from the Delaware Division of Substance Abuse and Mental Health. All other controlled substance prescribing utilizing telemedicine in Delaware is determined by reference to the same standards of care and practice as for prescribing following in-person encounters.[16]

Federal and State Fraud and Abuse Laws

Physicians considering entering into agreements with established telemedicine companies, telemedicine technology vendors, or healthcare facilities in order to render telemedicine services to facility patients may need to carefully consider compliance with federal fraud and abuse laws. Specifically, physicians should engage legal counsel to review the arrangement for compliance with the Anti-Kickback Statute and the Physician Self-Referral Law (commonly referred to as the Stark Law).

---

[16] 24 Del. Admin. Code § 19.2.

The Stark Law

The Stark Law prohibits a physician from referring Medicare or Medicaid beneficiaries for designated health services (DHS) to an entity with which the physician or immediate family member has a financial relationship, unless an exception applies.[17] It also prohibits the entity from submitting claims to Medicare or Medicaid for services resulting from a prohibited referral. The potential penalties are significant, including overpayment refund obligations, False Claims Act liability, civil monetary penalties, and exclusion from participation in federal healthcare programs.

The Stark Law applies only to the referral of DHS, which includes specifically defined items and services, including clinical laboratory services, physical and occupational therapy services, radiology and certain other imaging services, and durable medical equipment and supplies, among others. The financial relationships implicated by the Stark Law include both compensation arrangements and ownership/investment interests.

Common exceptions utilized in telemedicine arrangements include the rental of office space exception, the rental of equipment exception, bona fide employment relationships, personal service arrangements (applicable to independent contractor relationships), and the fair market value compensation exception, among others.

The Stark Law is often implicated where a physician rents office space or equipment from an entity to which the physician refers DHS. The Stark Law may also be implicated, for example, where a hospital engages and compensates a physician to render telemedicine services to hospital patients, or where a laboratory offers free telemedicine platform for the performance of telepathology, and where the physician may refer DHS to the hospital or laboratory.

Physicians should also consider whether the applicable state has a similar physician self-referral law. Delaware, for example, does not have a similar law.

---

[17] 42 U.S.C. § 1395nn.

Anti-Kickback Statute

The Anti-Kickback Statute makes it a criminal offense to knowingly and willfully offer, pay, solicit, or receive, directly or indirectly, anything of value in return for referring, furnishing, arranging for, or recommending items or services reimbursable by any federal healthcare program.[18] Unlike the Stark Law, the Anti-Kickback Statute does not require compliance with an exception or safe harbor to the law, although compliance is generally advisable. Like the Stark Law, there are common safe harbors to the Anti-Kickback Statute, including the space and equipment rental safe harbors, the bona fide employment relationship safe harbor, and the personal services and management contracts safe harbor.

The Anti-Kickback Statute may be implicated where a physician receives something of value in exchange for referrals of items or services reimbursed by a federal healthcare program. For example, if a health system leases equipment to a rural physician to expand availability to patients in such communities, the parties should consider compliance with a safe harbor to avoid allegations that the equipment is provided for less than fair market value in order to secure referrals to the health system. Physicians should also consider whether the applicable state has a similar Anti-Kickback Statute. Delaware, for example, does have an Anti-Kickback Statute that applies to referrals for items or services reimbursable by Delaware Medicaid.[19]

Conclusion

This chapter identifies common issues in telemedicine legal compliance. Additional issues also warrant consideration, including standards and requirements for reimbursement and health information privacy and security. Physicians should carefully consider these issues, and consider working with legal counsel, before establishing a practice via telemedicine or entering into an arrangement with a third party involving practice via telemedicine.

---

[18] 42 U.S.C. § 1320a-7b(b).

[19] 31 Del. Code §1005.

Ethical Concerns in Telemedicine

5

M. Wade Shrader

Telemedicine use is steadily increasing as a method of how patients access healthcare in the world today [1]. Common uses of telemedicine include applications to rural locations, routine health maintenance follow-up, and expanded access to subspecialty service [2].

Interest in telehealth for pediatric orthopedics, for example, is growing, as indicated by the 2017 Pediatric Orthopedic Society of North America (POSNA) membership survey on telehealth [3]. However, one of the largest concerns of the POSNA members was over the "ethical implications" of telehealth/telemedicine. No additional details were asked in this membership survey. However, there are several reports in the literature on the ethical issues in telehealth.

There are four basic principles of medical ethics which include Autonomy, Justice, Beneficence, and Nonmaleficence. Autonomy is considered the coercion-free decision-making patients have regarding their healthcare. Justice is defined as healthcare equity distributed among all groups in society. Beneficence underlies

M. W. Shrader (✉)
Department of Orthopedic Surgery, Nemours A.I. duPont Hospital for Children, Wilmington, DE, USA
e-mail: wade.shrader@nemours.org

© Springer Nature Switzerland AG 2021
A. Atanda Jr., J. F. Lovejoy III (eds.), *Telemedicine in Orthopedic Surgery and Sports Medicine*,
https://doi.org/10.1007/978-3-030-53879-8_5

that the healthcare service provided should be for the good of the patient and not for anyone else's primary benefit. And, finally Nonmaleficence dictates that the service does not harm the patient or others in society [4].

Certainly the basic tenets of medical ethics should be the foundation for any medicine that is practiced, including telemedicine. The importance of truth in physician and healthcare practice advertising is paramount [5–7]. However, the ethics of telemedicine also would include several aspects of the ethics of business practices inside the context of a medical practice. Those medical business ethics principles have evolved over recent decades. Explosion of social media amplifies the ethical implications of medical marketing given its widespread audience and extension essentially of the marketplace. Very few medical societies have created guidelines and policies on the ethical implications of these business practices.

There are several specific ethical issues that come about from the use of telemedicine and information technology (IT) health information. Langerizadeh et al. published a systematic review of 25 articles between 2012 and 2017 [8] that demonstrated concerns about technology and specifically how some aspects of patient populations may not have access to the appropriate technology to optimally access telehealth opportunities. This barrier to telemedicine would be a potential example of a violation of the Justice principle of medical ethics. Other concerns from the systematic review include loss of physician-patient physical contact, potential negative impacts to the informed consent process, and confidentiality/data issues.

Dr. David Fleming from the Missouri Center of Health Ethics has written extensively on the medical ethics of telemedicine with his research being focused on consent, confidentiality, and privacy. His 2009 article reported that privacy concerns were the primary issue from patients when seeking healthcare via an electronic means [9].

Although Fleming is an advocate for the expansion of telemedicine use throughout our healthcare ecosystem, he does not minimize the ethical issues either, noting that ensuring justice, access, and equity are all significant challenges. Ironically, as it's important to note, the very patients who may benefit the most from telemedicine services may not have the financial and technological means to access it [9].

The American College of Physicians (ACP) policy paper on telemedicine and primary care provides further views on medical ethics [2]. They clearly state that a valid patient-provider relationship must exist for a telemedicine service to take place. They state that the burden should be on the providers to confirm the identity of the patients even though they are seeing them through telemedicine encounters. They did state, however, that real-time audio and video technology could be used to establish such a relationship and that the physician should use his/her judgment for which patients would most best benefit from telemedicine and and should not sacrifice their ethical obligation for the sake of new technology.

The American Medical Association (AMA) also has a statement on the ethics of telemedicine and virtual encounters. In general, the principles are that physicians have the same duties to our patients in telemedicine encounters as we do during in-person encounters. Moreover, the physician-patient relationship should be maintained as the most important aspect of the relationship. Specifically, they state "the relationship between patient and physician is based on trust and gives rise to physicians' ethical obligations to place the patient's welfare above their own self-interest, and above obligations to other groups..." [10]. The AMA counsel on ethical and judicial affairs has had to position papers including that of Chaet et al. reported on the ethical practice of telehealth and telemedicine [11].

Shore et al. also reported on the AMA's counsel recommendations and use of social media [10].This report has several practical recommendations for the physician considering the use of telemedicine. These are listed below:

1. Inform patients of limitations of the therapeutic relationship.
2. Advise patients how to arrange follow-up if needed.
3. Encourage patients to inform their primary care physician of the online health encounter.
4. A telehealth provider should be proficient in the use of the relevant technology.

5. Telehealth providers should recognize the limitations of the relevant technology and take reasonable steps to overcome those (i.e., have someone else do a physical exam locally).

In particular the AMA Council on Ethical and Judicial Affairs recommends that physicians be prudent and carrying out a diagnostic evaluation. Elements of that prudence include every effort to establish the patient's identity, confirming that telemedicine is appropriate for this patient's needs, and evaluating the indications for any treatment. Finally the physician should document all aspects of the clinical evaluation similar to if it were an in-person encounter.

The informed consent process should also be tailored to reflect the telemedicine environment. The patient should have a clear understanding of how telemedicine works, the limitations of this method of evaluation, the credentials of the provider, and what is expected of the patients in this environment [12].

Expectations for continuity of care and the appropriate range of follow-up is a basic tenet of the ethical medical practice, which should be no different for telemedicine encounters. Providers should take steps to ensure continuity of care, discuss how follow-up will be arranged, and know how this information will be relayed back to the patient's primary care physician.

Finally, as telemedicine use cases continue to expand, the AMA encourages providers to support ongoing refinement of telemedicine practices. Physicians engaging in this type of digital health practice should advocate for policies and initiatives to improve telemedicine quality of care. The active telemedicine physician should also routinely monitor the digital health landscape to identify and address opportunities for improvement.

In conclusion, telemedicine can offer a great deal of quality services to our patients. The ethical practices of medicine that we have during in-person encounters should also be applied in all telemedicine encounters. The practical use of telemedicine is certainly in the ever-evolving healthcare landscape, and physicians should be savvy in that landscape in order to provide high-quality care and to practice good, ethical medicine.

References

1. Kim T, Zuckerman JE. Realizing the potential of telemedicine in global health. J Glob Health. 2019;9(2):020307.
2. Worth T. Telehealth: the balance between access and ethics. Med Econ. 2015;29:31.
3. Williams BA, Guerrero A, Blakemore LC, Frick SL. Surveying the POSNA landscape: what can we learn from society survey studies? J Pediatr Orthop. 2020;40(1):e63–7.
4. Siegler M, Pellegrino Edmund D, Singer PA. Clinical medical ethics. J Clin Ethic. 1990;1:5–9.
5. Smith CP, George D. When is advertising a plastic surgeon's individual "Brand" unethical? AMA J Ethics. 2018;20(4):372–8.
6. Powel R. The ethics of biomedical markets. J Med Ethics. 2015;41(6):431–2.
7. Fuster V. The hazards of physician advertising. J Am Coll Cardiol. 2015;66(22):2561–2.
8. Langarizadeh M, Moghbeli AA. Application of ethics for providing telemedicine services and information technology. Med Arch. 2017;71(5):351–5.
9. Fleming DA, Edison KE, Pak H. Telehealth ethics. Telemed J E Health. 2009;15(8):797–803.
10. Shore R, Halsy J, Shah K, Crigger BJ, Douglas SP. Report of the AMA council on ethical and judicial affairs; professionalism in the use of social medial. J Clin Ethics. 2011;22(2):165–72.
11. Chaet D, Clearfield SJE, Skimming K. Ethical practice in telehealth and telemedicine. J Gen Intern Med. 2017;32(10):1136–40.
12. Nelson WA. The ethics of telemedicine. Healthc Exec. 2010;25(6):50–3.

Section II

Telemedicine in Daily Use

Telemedicine Etiquette

6

Tina Gustin

Telemedicine requires professionals to develop the patient-professional relationship in a different and more deliberate manner [1]. One can be an excellent in-person provider but fail as a telemedicine provider. There is a unique and different skill set required for this type of encounter [2]. Providers spend countless hours learning how to demonstrate empathy, provide motivational interviewing, and read body language for in-person visits. They are not, however, trained in methods to translate these skills into a telemedicine encounter. Unfortunately, most medical schools are not preparing future physicians for this type of visit. In addition, most companies that sell telemedicine technologies are not preparing providers for this type of delivery. The education that most telemedicine vendors deliver addresses only how to correctly and safely use the equipment, security, and how to troubleshoot technical issues. The unique interpersonal skills or human factors necessary for a successful telemedicine visit do not intuitively "flip" from the traditional in-person skill set.

Human factor science is concerned with understanding the interactions among humans and other elements of a system such

T. Gustin (✉)
Old Dominion University, Norfolk, VA, USA
e-mail: tgustin@odu.edu

as telemedicine [3]. In telemedicine, there is a need to make sure the users can overcome the barriers imposed by technology in a manner that allows for projection of respect, empathy, appropriate communication, and satisfactory interactions for both the provider and patients. Learning how to connect with a patient and display empathy is a skill that all providers must be able to display regardless of the delivery format. Learning how to project this virtually is a skill that is the key to success as a telemedicine provider. These unique human factor skills have been coined "telehealth etiquette."

While most providers use social media platforms such as FaceTime, Skype, and text messaging to communicate with family and friends, this informal approach can lead to lazy or unprofessional use of similar professional platforms. Unfortunately, this social use does not translate into a telemedicine encounter. The casual nature of social platforms has led to disinhibited behaviors such as diminished empathy and disinterested expressions. This disinhibited behavior is diminished regardless of age, gender, or profession. It has been suggested that this everyday use of technology has lessened individual's abilities to empathize and pick up on nonverbal cues when using technology to communicate [4]. This type of casual communication should not be replicated with telemedicine.

Defining Telehealth Etiquette

Telehealth etiquette can be thought of as the soft skills or "screen side etiquette" unique to the telemedicine encounter. Telehealth etiquette includes both verbal and nonverbal expressions from the provider. It includes the environment and privacy considerations unique to a virtual encounter. This type of visit must be conducted in a different and deliberate manner from that of a traditional in-person visit. Many telemedicine failures have not occurred because of failed equipment but because of poor etiquette and failed performance [5]. Telemedicine technology is important, but without proper relationship building, telemedicine is not going to work [5]. Patient satisfaction with telemedicine hinges on the communication with the provider, not the technology or physical presence [6].

When considering telehealth etiquette, there are three distinct categories that must be addressed. They include (1) environment, (2) privacy, and (3) performance. A telemedicine encounter is optimized in situations where these three categories are addressed enabling distractors to be removed. The provider should take time to address each of these issues prior to and during the virtual visit.

Telehealth Categories

Environment

Visual factors can enhance the telemedicine encounter allowing the patient to focus on the provider during the telemedicine visit. The *provider's appearance* must be carefully considered. A professional appearance should be maintained for all encounters. To assure this professional appearance, several simple techniques should be maintained for all visits. Clothing choices should be carefully considered for the virtual visit. Dark colors should be avoided as they will wash out the appearance of the provider. Patterns such as herringbone, stripes, and busy prints should also be avoided as they may appear as wavy lines or a blur on the screen which is distracting for the patient [7]. Glittery jewelry may appear as a flash on screen and should be avoided. Ideally providers should wear a lab coat for all telemedicine encounters. The traditional lab coat will not only provide a professional appearance but will cover any distracting color or print the provider may be wearing.

Movements that are not generally noticed during an in-person visit such as pushing glasses up, brushing hair behind the ears, or talking with one's hands are amplified on the video screen. These simple everyday movements become annoying distractors during telemedicine encounters. The analogy is the difference between stage acting and television acting. The in-person visit is the stage actor. Large movements and intonations are necessary in this setting. The telemedicine visit is the television actor. In this setting, subtle movements and gestures and a quieter intonation appear much larger on the screen [8].

The appearance of the location or *room setting* that the provider has selected to conduct the virtual visit from is just as important as their personal appearance. The telehealth room or setting must be prepared for the visit. Some providers may prefer a fold-out screen with their facilities' name or logo imprinted on the screen. This type of background, while not necessary, assures a consistent professional background. At a minimum, the room or setting should appear neat and as professional as possible. Desks should be cleared from paper, books, backpacks, or other distracting items. Office clutter will divert the patient's focus from the provider. Food and drinks should be removed prior to the visit. Objects in the background should be assessed prior to a visit recognizing that pictures on the wall will be in full view. Providers should consider removing any political or possible controversial posters or art. The most desirable wall color for telehealth is a medium blue or gray color. The wall paint should be flat based to avoid reflection.

The *lighting* in the room is critical. Natural light works best for all skin tones, but unfortunately this type of light source is not found in most healthcare facilities. A bright open window behind the provider will turn them into a shadowed silhouette [9, 10]. Placing a lamp in front of you often provides the best light for patients to be able to read nonverbal cues. Mixing light sources such as LED and fluorescent lighting will affect the image quality. Mixed lighting can cause a flickering effect. It is important that the provider runs several tests before beginning a visit to assure that the light source and camera position work.

Noises that are overlooked during an in-person visit serve as distractors for telemedicine visits. The providers should make themselves aware of things that will produce distracting background noises [11, 12]. Telemedicine microphones are very sensitive and can pick up sounds such as typing, jewelry clanking on the desk, the clicking of a pen, or the rustling of paper. Chewing gum can produce distracting sounds and even make the provider's words unclear. Multiple providers in a visit must avoid any side conversations or taking phone calls.

Background noises in the area of the visit can also produce a distraction. Such distractions might include office chatter, traffic, the ringing of phones, overhead announcements, and beepers. In order to minimize external noises, the provider will want to (1) shut the door, (2) inform those at your site of the telehealth visit, (3) put a sign on the door informing others that a telehealth visit is taking place, (5) select a room that is removed from active areas, and (6) turn off or mute the phones/mute pagers.

The provider must be sure to speak clearly and maintain an even volume when speaking. One must always assume the audio is on and be sure to not say anything that you would not want a patient to hear. It is a best practice to mute the microphone when not speaking.

Privacy

Issues surrounding patient privacy, confidentiality, and legal regulations have created barriers for the adoption of telemedicine as well [13]. Both providers and patients have concerns about the confidentiality of health information being transmitted through the Internet and cloud-based technology [14]. Fears over unauthorized access and the decoding of the encrypted information have prevented both patients and healthcare providers from openly engaging in the use of telemedicine [13].

Protecting a patient's privacy during a telemedicine encounter brings a different set of challenges. During an in-person visit, the door would be closed, video recordings would not occur, and everyone in the room would be seen and identified. During a telemedicine encounter, the provider will need to take additional steps to assure that privacy matters are addressed. The provider should never assume that the video equipment is off. The equipment should always be checked prior to the visit, the lens cover should be in place, and the audio should be on mute to avoid accidental HIPAA violations prior to the start of a visit. If the provider is conducting the visit from a busy office space, headphones should be considered instead of loud computer speakers; this will avoid protected health information from being heard outside of the office.

At the start of every encounter, the provider should assure that the patient is in a secure area. The provider should ask the patient to identify anyone in the room. It is often helpful to have the patient move the camera around the room to allow the provider the opportunity to see the setting and people with the patient. The provider may want to do the same for their space. Most telemedicine platforms are designed to prevent patients from recording an encounter; the provider should check for this feature when platforms are selected. Many telemedicine consents now state that recordings will not occur and request that the patient does not record the session either. Most states now require that a consent for the telemedicine encounter is signed prior to the visit; this should always be checked prior to the encounter.

Performance

The provider's performance is key to a successful visit. Poor verbal and nonverbal communication, inappropriate utilization of equipment, and not being prepared for the visit may derail the most experienced in-person provider. Research has consistently demonstrated that patient satisfaction is dependent on the perception of how the providers communicate [15]. An effective patient-centered interview that is well paced, utilizes open-ended questions, and allows the patient time to respond without interruptions is key to any type of visit whether in person or virtual. This type of pacing is often difficult for new users to telemedicine. The screen may become the elephant in the room. Rather than beginning the visit with a relationship building discussion, the inexperienced telemedicine provider often rushes through the visit forgetting the key elements of the encounter.

Timing, pacing, and small talk must be purposeful. At the start of the encounter, the providers should not only introduce themselves but tell the patient a little about themselves. They should let the patient know what to expect from the telemedicine visit. If this is not done at the start of the encounter, the whole appointment will feel distant and mechanical.

The provider must make every effort to provide *eye contact* and create facial expression that enhance the provider-patient relationship. Appropriate eye gaze displays empathy and genuine concern to the patient [16]. Proper camera placement will allow the provider to shift their eye gaze downward while still appearing to be looking at the patient. Placing a camera on the top of the computer screen will allow for a certain amount of gaze angle that the patient will not notice. When the camera is placed closer to eye level and the provider's eyes gazes downward, the provider will appear to be looking downward and not at the patient [16]. Humans generally cannot perceive a downward gaze angle of less than 5–7 degrees [17]. A simple formula to achieve the 5–7 degree gaze angle is to position the chair 4–6 feet from the camera [16].

Providers should also let the patient know when they are looking down or to the side for charting. Without this situational awareness, patients often perceive this eye gaze and head tilt as disinterest. Head placement in the screen is critical. The provider should assure at the start of the visit that their upper body and head are placed in the center of the screen. Too often the top of a provider's head is "cut off." While it is important to check placement, it is equally important to not continue to check one's appearance in the small block on the screen that allows the providers to "check themselves." Many providers have a habit of checking themselves throughout the visit.

Some providers may also portray a "resting face" during the visit. A resting face is the facial expression most often made by individuals when not speaking. The resting face is the most powerful nonverbal form of communication [18]. The resting face for a telemedicine provider is amplified and can be interpreted as disinterest or disagreement. Often the resting face and verbal interaction are incongruent. The providers should know their resting face and develop strategies to check themselves during the visit. Simple strategies such as checking in with one's self in a mirror, recording yourself, or asking a friend or peer what their resting face is will help the provider to "know" their resting face [18]. Maintaining congruence between facial and verbal communication is critical.

The provider should be sure to not interrupt the conversation with the patient. There is sometimes a video delay that could cause both the patient and provider to talk over each other. Because of this feature, the provider must practice active listening and repeat back what the patient has said so that they feel understood and validated. Another consideration is the effective use of pauses. Periods of active listening and quiet are effective for an in-person visit but feel like awkward long periods of silence in telemedicine visits.

While the importance of *empathy* in patient care is well documented in healthcare literature, it is not similarly addressed with regard to telehealth [19]. Some studies have suggested that empathetic gestures and utterances are less evident in telemedicine consultations [20]. A significant portion of the in-person visit tends to be nonverbal (body language, tone of voice), and without these cues, providers may not be able to read and respond to their patients' needs appropriately. Empathy, often delivered by touch from many providers in the traditional in-person encounter, is more difficult to provide during a telemedicine encounter. Other modes of expression must be used to convey empathy. Telemedicine providers must consciously lean into the camera, nod, and assure that they are maintaining good eye contact. Purposeful words of understanding and concern are also more vital when touch is not an option [11, 19].

The provider's performance with the *telemedicine equipment* may also be disruptive. For instance, if the provider is unsure how to use some of the telemedicine settings, the provider may lose credibility, and the patient may become less interested in participating in telemedicine. It is thus important for the provider to practice with the equipment before the encounter and if needed have someone nearby that can address telemedicine equipment issues if they occur.

The provider must also come to the telemedicine visit *prepared* with any necessary notes, test results, referral information, or care plans. It is disconcerting for a patient to feel as though the provider has no understanding of their health issues. Prior to a telemedicine session, it is imperative for the provider to obtain the needed records, review them, and consult with other providers as indicated. This will allow the session to run smoother and the outcomes to be optimized.

The closure of the telemedicine visit is an important as the beginning. New telemedicine providers often end the visit abruptly. The provider should not end the appointment quickly by turning the camera off. They must be sure to leave time for questions and answers at the end of the session. There are many checklists available to providers that are designed to assist them with a successful telemedicine encounter. See telemedicine visit checklist (Table 6.1) and telemedicine etiquette checklist (Table 6.2).

Table 6.1 Telemedicine visit checklist

Pre-telehealth event checklist	Check
1. Check equipment	
2. Check environment for clutter and distracting items	
3. Check clothing, and get lab coat	
4. Mute phone and pager	
5. Assure the patient has signed the Telehealth Consent form and has an opportunity to ask questions or be provided with additional information	
6. The patient has an opportunity to request an interpreter or other support to enable maximum benefit of the encounter	
7. A backup communication plan (telephone, etc.) is developed and communicated to provider	
8. Share provider and patient alternative contact information	
9. Place a Telehealth In-Session sign on the door	
10. Assure that both the patient and provider's sites are secure	
At the start of the visit	
1. Assure the patients know that the visit will be virtual	
2. Check that patient's setting is secure	
3. Seating should be checked to assure full visibility	
4. Assess for proper lighting and adjust as needed	
5. Place camera at the same elevation as the eyes (when possible)	
6. Assure that the face is clearly visible	
7. Begin visit with relationship building questions "small talk"	
During the visit	
1. Assure that patient is not recording visit	
2. Identify yourself when you speak (if there are multiple providers)	
3. Speak clearly with a strong voice	
4. Use meaningful empathetic word choices	
5. Avoid long periods of silence	
6. Allow for audio delay	
7. Allow time for questions	
8. Avoid interrupting others; give a visual cue for who should speak next	
9. Let the patient know if you are charting and looking down	

Reprinted with permission Tina Gustin 12/31/19

Table 6.2 Telemedicine etiquette checklist

Etiquette categories	Requirements	Check

Appearance	Well groomed
	Lab coat when appropriate
	Visible badge to identify self
	Choose clothing
	  -Not dark
	  -Limited in patterns
	  -No glitter
	Limit jewelry
	  -No bangles or dangling jewelry
	  -Minimal jewelry	

Distractors	Make sure equipment functioning (check 15 minutes prior) Minimize outside noise Remove clutter from room No eating or drinking Shut door and put sign up regarding meeting Let others know telehealth visit is taking place Assess lighting (both provider and patient sides) Limit paper shuffling, pen tapping, etc. Limit quick body and hand movements Mute microphone when not in use Turn off pagers and phones	
Privacy	Assess security of environments Introduce everyone in room (provider and patient side) Determine if patient would like to proceed Show room with camera Assure patient of equipment security Do not record meeting	

Nonverbal communication	Look at camera and not patient's face on screen
	Check provider view screen
	  -Eye contact
	  -Position of body in picture
	  -Distractors
	Minimize gestures
	Use facial expressions to express emotions
	Minimize charting	

Table 6.2 (continued)

Etiquette categories	Requirements	Check
Verbal communication	Use words to convey thoughts Use motivational interviewing Limit dead space	
Empathy	Lean in Use words to express empathy Nod Maintain eye contact	

Reprint by permission Tina Gustin 12/31/19

Telemedicine Visits Any Time, But Not Anywhere

Where not to conduct a telemedicine visit may sound simple, experienced telemedicine providers have reported less than secure locations for telemedicine visits. The ease of use and quick access will afford the busy orthopedic surgeon the ability to complete a consultation anytime, but not necessarily anywhere. Currently telemedicine policies do not regulate where a provider site can and cannot be. The ideal location for a telemedicine visit is a dedicated space. This space can be in a provider's office or home. As discussed earlier, this will ensure privacy, proper lighting and audio, and avoid interruptions. Unfortunately, experienced providers have reported conducting visits in the grocery store, restaurants, bars, and parties. One suggestion for the on-call provider would be to pack their badge and lab coat when heading out. Consults that occur away from work or home can be taken in a quiet secure area or a parked car. Providers should only take these on-the-spot consultations with a secure device and platform. Currently popular platforms such as FaceTime and Skype are not considered HIPAA secure. At the start of these "anywhere" visits, the provider should make the patient aware of their location.

Common Provider Errors

While many of the strategies discussed seem common sense, experienced telemedicine providers as well as new users tend to make the same mistakes. Listed below are common behaviors observed in practice:

- Forgetting to check equipment prior to the visit
- Not muting the microphone
- Conducting visits in areas that are not secure
- Not checking the background
- Looking down and appearing to be disinterested
- Incongruent facial expressions and word choices
- Inability to emote empathy
- Missed parts of the telemedicine visit such as the relationship building or closure
- Distracting behaviors (fidgeting with glasses and hair)
- Not centering the face in the screen
- Eating and drinking during the visit

Stories from the Field of Telemedicine

To illustrate the errors that occur regularly in the telemedicine industry, you will find below sampling mistakes that experienced telemedicine providers have made. These stories have been taken from providers that have shared their stories openly at telehealth conferences and meetings. While some may be funny, they are intended to demonstrate how small errors can have big consequences.

HIPAA Breach

An on-call neurologist took a telemedicine stroke call in the middle of the night. He began the telemedicine consult from a secure laptop located in his bedroom. As he was examining the patient and directing them to raise their arms to touch their nose, he asked "can you see me." The immediate response from the provider at the remote site was "yes doctor we can see you and the person in bed behind you." The doctor had gotten out of bed in his bedroom without checking his surroundings or attire. His partner could be seen in the bed behind him by both the patient and provider. He had also forgotten to put a shirt on and was conducting the visit topless.

Break in Professionalism

Another interesting story is about an orthopedic surgeon that had been conducting telehealth visits for years. His comfort with technology and desire to evaluate patients anytime anywhere led to an informal approach to care. With his increasing comfort, he began to take telemedicine calls from restaurants and bars. While he did go to a quiet corner to conduct the visit on the setting, he was clearly not conducting the visits in a HIPAA secure space for the visit.

Cluttered Environment

An experienced telemedicine psychiatrist was conducting a telemedicine visit with an established pediatric client diagnosed with a paranoid personality disorder. As the visit progressed, it was apparent that the child was becoming more and more agitated. Finally, the child jumped up, slammed his chair down, and yelled "You have a tree growing out your head and you are not paying attention to me." The provider had not assessed his office background. He had a beautiful house plant behind his desk. Indeed, it looked like he had plant growing from his head. He was also looking down charting giving this young man the appearance of disinterest. This family did not elect to continue using telehealth for their counseling appointments.

Not Checking Equipment

A primary care provider had not muted the computer's microphone prior to a follow-up telemedicine visit. As the patient's information was handed to the provider by the medical assistant, he stated "I don't know why this patient continues to make appointments. She does not follow directions or have her medications filled. This is a waste of time for both of us." The patient was already online and heard the comment. She did not complete the virtual visit and did not return to the provider for care.

Lack of Empathy

A surgeon was evaluating a teenage patient following a surgical procedure for a skeletal deformity. During the virtual assessment, the child was tearful and stated "I really do not like the way that my chest looks. I wish I had never had this surgery." The surgeon was uncomfortable with the encounter. Instead of saying "I am sorry that you feel that way, tell me what you do not like about the way your chest looks," the surgeon rushed through that part of the visit. She felt unable to provide empathetic feedback; as a result, the child's feelings were not explored or validated. The surgeon moved quickly through the assessment without opening the door for the patient to further express concerns.

While these stories seem extreme, they are real. It is critical that the simple steps reviewed in this chapter are followed.

Conclusion

It should not be assumed that just because a person is an experienced in-person provider, they will be able to deliver the same care via telemedicine without training. Preparing a provider for the unique skills required for telemedicine etiquette will pay great dividends in both patient and provider satisfaction with the delivery of care. It is only through a conscious understanding and awareness of how the telemedicine encounter differs from the in-person visit that the provider will be able to create a sense of presence where both the patient and provider forget that the visit is occurring virtually. This is only possible when the provider has the needed skills for this type of encounter.

References

1. Rienitis H, Teuss G, Bonney AD. Teaching telehealth consulting skills. Clin Teach. 2016;13(2):119–23.
2. Miller EA. The technical and interpersonal aspects of telemedicine: Effects on doctor patient communication. J Telemed Telecare. 2003;9(1):1–7.

3. Demiris G, Charness N, Krupinski E, Ben-Arieh D, Washington K, Wu J, et al. The role of human factors in telehealth. Telemed J E Health. 2010;16(4):446–53. https://doi.org/10.1089/tmj.2009.0114.

4. Konrath SH, O'Brien EH, Hsing C. Changes in dispositional empathy in American college students over time: A meta-analysis. Personal Soc Psychol Rev. 2011;15(2):180–98.

5. Laff M. [Internet] American Academy of Family Physicians; 2014. Telemedicine can build bridge to expand health care, say panelist. 2014 Feb 5 [cited 2020, Jan 1];[about 1 page] Available from: https://www.aafp.org/news/practice-professional-issues/20140205rgctelemedicineforum.html?_ga=2.193455087.314442142.1577888644-839054758.1577888644

6. Heath S. [Internet] Patient EngagmentHIT; What are patient preferences for technology, provider communication? 2019 March 12 [cited 2020, Jan 1];[about 1 page] Available from: https://patientengagementhit.com/news/what-are-patient-preferences-for-technology-provider-communication

7. Calm P. [Internet] Polycom; Make video conferencing great for all great tips from Polly Calm, the world's expert in vidiquette. 2016 [cited 2020, Jan 1];[about 10 screens] Available from: https://www.polycom.com/hd-video-conferencing/polly-calm-vidiquette.html

8. Master Class [Internet] Master Class; Helen Mirren's top film acting tips. Master Class. 2019 [cited 2020, Jan 1];[about 5 min]Available from: https://www.masterclass.com/articles/helen-mirrens-top-film-acting-tips?utm_source=Paid&utm_medium=Bing

9. Carroll TB. [Internet] Rural Health Quarterly; Four keys to telemedicine etiquette. 2018 Sept 5 [cited 2020, Jan 1];[about 1 screen]. Available from: http://ruralhealthquarterly.com/home/2018/09/05/four-keys-to-telemedicine-etiquette/

10. Wade E. [Internet] Barton Associates; Tips for telemedicine care: prepping your virtual exam room. 2018 June 28 [cited 2020 Jan 1]; [about 1 screen]. Available from: https://www.bartonassociates.com/blog/tips-for-telemedicine-care-prepping-your-virtual-exam-room

11. Edelson C. [blog on the Internet] 2017 Feb 6 [cited 2019 Dec 20] In: PCC pediatric EHR [Internet] solutions virtual bedside manner: connecting with telemedicine. Solutions. Available from: https://blog.pcc.com/virtual-bedside-manner-connecting-with-telemedicine

12. Major J. [Internet] Arizona Telemedicine Program. Using telemediquette to make your telemedicine encounters effective. 2016 Nov 17 [cited 2020 Jan 1]; [about 1 screen] . Available from: https://telemedicine.arizona.edu/blog/using-telemediquette-make-your-telemedicine-encounters-effective

13. Doarn CR. The last challenges and barriers to the development of telemedicine programs. Stud Health Technol Inform. 2008;131:45–54.

14. Brennan DM, Baker LM. Human factors in the development and implementation of telerehabilitation systems. J Telemed Telecare. 2008;14:55–8.

15. Berman AC, Chutka DS. Assessing effective physician-patient communication skills: "Are you listing to me doc?". Kor J Med Educ. 2016;28(2):243–9.
16. Chen M. Leveraging the asymmetric sensitivity of eye contact for video-conference. In: Proceedings of the CHI Proceedings of the SIGHI conference on human factors in computing systems. Minneapolis: ACM Press; 2002. p. 49–56. Available at: https://dl.acm.org/doi/10.1145/503376.503386.
17. American Telemedicine Association. [Internet] A concise guide for telemedicine practitioners: human factors quick guide eye contact. 2018 Oct 3 [cited 2019 Dec 1]; [about 1 page]. Available from: https://www.americantelemed.org/resources/a-concise-guide-for-telemedicine-practitioners-human-factors-quick-guide-eye-contact/
18. Guarino J. [Internet] Institute of Public Speaking; 2019. Know your resting face. [cited 2020 Jan 1];[about 1 screen] Available from: https://www.instituteofpublicspeaking.com/know-resting-face/
19. Terry C, Cain J. The emerging issue of digital empathy. Am J Pharm Educ. 2016;80(4):58. https://doi.org/10.5688/ajpe80458.
20. Liu X, Sawada Y. Doctor-patient communication: a comparison between telemedicine consultation and face-to-face consultation. Intern Med. 2007;46(5):227–32.

Virtual Musculoskeletal Examination Using Telemedicine

7

Alfred Atanda Jr. and Suken A. Shah

One of the biggest barriers to adoption of telemedicine from the perspective of orthopedic care providers is concern about the ability to do an adequate physical examination. Orthopedic surgeons feel the physical exam is of utmost importance when formulating a differential diagnosis and appropriate treatment plan. However, there are also many situations where a "virtual" physical examination may be enough to appropriately treat a patient. Many established patients that we see in person present for a wound check after surgery, to review medical imaging, and for surveillance exam to ensure that he/she is progressing along the treatment plan or discuss a surgical procedure. In these scenarios, a detailed, thorough physical examination may not be necessary. When seeing new patients, we often use telemedicine to not definitively diagnose and treat them, but more as a screening tool to determine if and when an in-person visit is needed (and with whom) and also to order appropriate imaging beforehand. There are many tips and tricks that one can utilize to ensure that the virtual physical examination is as valuable as possible and that the experience is efficient and rewarding for both parties involved. We have found it useful to make a one-page "tip" sheet that the

A. Atanda Jr. (✉) · S. A. Shah
Department of Orthopedic Surgery, Nemours/Alfred I. duPont Hospital for Children, Wilmington, DE, USA
e-mail: aatanda@nemours.org; sshah@nemours.org

© Springer Nature Switzerland AG 2021
A. Atanda Jr., J. F. Lovejoy III (eds.), *Telemedicine in Orthopedic Surgery and Sports Medicine*,
https://doi.org/10.1007/978-3-030-53879-8_7

81

patient receives prior to the telemedicine visit to outline the specific provider's preferences.

Prior to the Virtual Visit

A common barrier to an effective orthopedic physical examination is an inability to see the patient's entire body or limbs in a functional range of motion. Many patients simply present to the virtual visit dressed in casual clothes sitting in front of the family computer at a desk. We have to ensure that we can see and evaluate the patient effectively; therefore, the patient should be in a place with ample room to walk, sit, lie down, and move their extremities freely. There should be ample lighting in order to visualize the patient appropriately. Back lighting (such as a bright window) should be avoided as much as possible as this can make it difficult to see cutaneous details, wounds, lacerations, erythema, or ecchymosis that require foreground lighting and the ability to see contrast. The patient should wear clothing that facilitates examination of the body area in question. Background noise, interference from pets, and other family members should be kept to a minimum. The patient should ensure that the interface device is appropriately charged and has a good Wi-Fi signal and that the patient is comfortable navigating the telemedicine app. (If possible, have an IT specialist from your organization review this with them prior to the visit.) The patient should ensure that he/she has any assistive ambulatory devices nearby to help with ambulation. Braces or orthoses should be readily available to check for fit and troubleshoot problems. Any dressings should be removed just prior to the visit to promote efficient examination. It may be helpful to have a family member or friend available to hold/maneuver the mobile device while the patient ambulates or performs range-of-motion exercises.

General Examination and Appearance

There are many things to note and document pertaining to the overall appearance of the patient. Just by interacting briefly with them, you can assess if they are alert and oriented, have appropriate affect, and are well-developed, well-nourished, and in no acute distress. You can visualize wounds/body areas for skin color/changes, swelling/effusion, drainage, lacerations, or presence of a rash. The patient or a family member can palpate an area for an assessment of tenderness. Also, this person can provide resistance with motion to get a vague sense of strength. Light touch/sensation can be assessed in a similar manner. Sitting posture and standing balance are evaluated easily.

Lower Extremity

Ask the patient to walk toward and away from the camera to demonstrate any gait disturbance or abnormality. Observing stance can demonstrate pelvic obliquity, genu varum/valgus, pes planus, or other alignment differences from the hip to the ankle. Knee range of motion in terms of flexion/extension, flexion contracture, or extensor lag can be assessed with the patient lying flat on a couch, bed, or floor. Ankle plantarflexion and dorsiflexion range can be assessed. Hip range of motion can be difficult, but forward flexion and abduction can be assessed while lying down. Watching for the ability to squat, do a straight-leg raise, and walk on the tiptoes/heels is an excellent way to assess strength. The patient or family member can squeeze his/her calf to assess calf tenderness.

Upper Extremity

Shoulder range of motion could be tested in terms of forward flexion, elevation, and abduction. Elbow range of motion in terms of flexion/extension, flexion contracture, or extensor lag can be assessed. Forearm supination/pronation and wrist flexion/extension can be assessed as well. Observing the patient making a fist, raising the thumb, abducting/adducting the digits, or making an "ok" sign is an easy way to assess nerve function. We find it effective, especially with children, so ask them to mirror our movements on their screen to quickly assess range of motion and function of the upper extremity and to elicit asymmetry.

Neck and Back

Neck rotation, tilt, flexion, and extension can be easily assessed in the virtual world, as well as most aspects of the cranial nerve and cervical dermatome exam, even provocative maneuvers with many cooperative patients. We advocate for neckless garments such as tank tops for these exams. For the thoracic and lumbar spine, we ask patients to dress in garments that show a maximum amount of the shoulders, trunk, and back to facilitate the virtual exam. Young children and males can simply be shirtless. Adolescents and young women have several options that work well: a zip-up hoodie/jacket or robe worn backward so the opening will allow a proper examination or a sports bra. Alignment of the patient's shoulders, scapulae, trunk, skin folds, waist, and pelvis can be quickly evaluated in the standing position; and trunk rotation and spine flexion can be assessed by forward bending away from the camera. Lateral bending, flexion, and extension can be easily assessed, and any maneuvers that reproduce pain can be recorded. Balance, gait, coordination, and strength can be assessed as mentioned above. Cutaneous malformations, skin abrasions, incisions, and swelling can all be assessed with good lighting.

Development and Implementation of Telemedicine in Practice

8

R. Michael Greiwe and Alfred Atanda Jr.

We now live in a world that futurist David Houle coined the "Shift Age", where older ideas and processes have been replaced by new technologies and innovations [1]. Some markets have more easily transformed their processes and ideas to the information age, while others changed more gradually. Standard mail was replaced by e-mail, Blockbuster gave way to Netflix, Ford gave up ground to Tesla, and JC Penney closed its doors to online marketplaces like Amazon and Wayfair. The online and mobile environment has become the new way of doing business, and product logistics, supply chain, and delivery are more critical than ever because speed and convenience are paramount to almost everything else.

In healthcare, change has come more gradually. Convenience is important to the consumer, but trust is also important. In today's competitive marketplaces, the locally trusted physician (especially orthopedic surgeon) has the upper hand over the mobile and digital telemedicine threats. What is clear in these environments is

R. M. Greiwe
Shoulder, Elbow and Sports Medicine, OrthoLive, CEO and OrthoCincy,
Edgewood, KY, USA
e-mail: mikegriewe@ortholive.com

A. Atanda Jr. (✉)
Department of Orthopedic Surgery, Nemours/Alfred I. duPont Hospital
for Children, Wilmington, DE, USA
e-mail: aatanda@nemours.org

© Springer Nature Switzerland AG 2021
A. Atanda Jr., J. F. Lovejoy III (eds.), *Telemedicine in Orthopedic
Surgery and Sports Medicine*,
https://doi.org/10.1007/978-3-030-53879-8_8

that those businesses who work with the consumer, and not against them, will be at a major competitive advantage over their peers.

The competitive landscape across urban populations has dictated a more rapid increase in telemedicine use among practices and physicians in urban populations. Innovative differentiators like telemedicine are being used as marketing tactics across the board.

We now live in a mobile world where the vast majority of Americans own a cell phone (96%) and 81% have a smartphone, up from 31% in 2011. Smartphone ownership is especially prevalent in the younger demographics, including those younger than 50 [2]. Physicians and medical staff are also increasingly reliant on cell phones to do their work and communicate with patients [3]. Research demonstrates that patients are not willing to be on hold for more than 2 minutes. Interestingly, the older patients are the less they are willing to wait on hold [4]. Average wait times at a large orthopedic practice in Cincinnati, Ohio, are more than 2 minutes. Over one in three patients is actually unwilling to call back after a long hold time [4]. This indicates that patients must be connected to your practice over their cell phones and that they would rather be contacted via text, rather than phone calls. Phone calls are viewed as intrusive to most younger adults, according to a study performed by OpenMarket.com [5]. According to a report published by Zendesk, customers feel the most satisfied when they can get their questions answered using a live chat feature, compared to options such as voice (88%), e-mail (85%), and even social media messaging (Facebook 84%, Twitter 77%) [6]. While medical questions probably shouldn't be answered via this mechanism, it points to the importance of HIPAA-secure chat features as we look to interact with our patients.

Telemedicine and app-based communication with our patients allows access to care for specialists and can decrease preventable complications and hospitalizations of patients who have poor access to care [7]. Access isn't the only thing that telemedicine does to benefit patients however. Cost and time savings were found for patients and providers in a study by Atanda et al. with orthopedic patients [8].

Simultaneously, our physicians are under tremendous practice pressures. Burnout and suicide rates among physicians are at all-time highs [9, 10]. In fact, physician suicide is double the rate of the general population and represents a higher rate than other professions, including the military [11]. Drivers of this epidemic are largely rooted within healthcare organizations which include excessive workloads and inefficient work processes. Given patient volume is unlikely to decline, efficiency is critically important to improve physician happiness and fulfillment.

Unfortunately, previous technology "advancements" in the form of electronic health records (EHRs) have contributed to the administrative burden and increased daily inefficiencies of physicians' practices. Most physicians spend over half of their time during a 10-hour workday with their EHR [12]. According to a recent study from Stanford University, seven in ten physicians disagree that their EHR has strengthened their patient relationships [13]. Most realistic measurements demonstrate that physicians lost approximately 20% productivity during the switch from written to electronic records. Even 2 years later, a study published by researchers from Drexel University in the *Journal of the Medical Informatics Association* demonstrated persistent productivity issues following EHR implementation [14].

However, it appears that telemedicine potentially can improve efficiencies for providers allowing them to see more patients in a smaller amount of time with less practice overhead compared to traditional visits [8, 15]. In addition, telehealth laws are changing, allowing physicians to see patients more easily and be reimbursed for their visits. For example, all private payers in parity states are required to reimburse for telemedicine visits. Coding for visits is becoming more simplified as well, opening the door for telemedicine to be utilized in a more mainstream way.

Competitive virtual practices are taking patients away from traditional brick-and-mortar practices because of their convenience and ability to perform medical care in a low overhead environment. This is most prevalent currently in primary care, where traditional visits can be more easily replaced with virtual visits. In orthopedics, postoperative visits, post-imaging visits, post-injection visits, and presurgical visits can be easily conducted via telemedicine. In addition, second-opinion consultation is especially being utilized with patients with orthopedic issues.

As a result, medical practices are coming to the realization that telemedicine can help them better meet the needs of their patients. In particular, it allows primary care and specialist physicians to be present in remote locations where access to their services has been traditionally limited. Probably most enticing, efficiency of virtual visits, especially in orthopedics, allows for providers to maximize their time. In addition, CEOs and practice administrators find that virtual care creates new pathways for patients to find the practice and new business models, including virtual urgent cares and worker's compensation evaluations.

Starting Your Telemedicine Practice

Asynchronous vs Synchronous Telemedicine

A critical component of understanding how to best utilize telemedicine in your practice is first understanding the different types of telemedicine and how each can benefit your practice.

Asynchronous telemedicine is a text, image, and video transmission that is in a "store-and-forward" type of environment. The easiest way to visualize this is to think of how we communicate over text messaging. This is asynchronous communication. Synchronous telemedicine is *live video-based communication*. Most telemedicine visits hosted today are in the form of synchronous visits. Asynchronous visits are not reimbursed as well in all states, and therefore, synchronous visits are most likely to be utilized. One important visit that can be utilized with asynchronous communication is postoperative visits. These visits lend themselves to asynchronous communication because photographs may be transmitted to understand how incisions appear.

Critical System Components

When choosing a telemedicine vendor, several important features must be met to ensure that your staff and providers as well as your patients have a seamless experience. First, a mobile application must be present for Mac and Android devices. Those that rely on web-based browsers are not proper for today's patients and require the patient to be tied to a computer or desk and a Wi-Fi signal, which is not ideal in today's world.

Second, there should be both a mobile and web applications for providers. Providers must be able to access their patients both on their mobile devices and during office hours from their desktop. Therefore, a web application is critically important for growth of your telemedicine business.

Third, especially in fields such as orthopedics and other surgical subspecialties that are dependent on imaging and laboratory follow-up, there must be an ability to provide screen sharing or image integration so that patients may be able to see as they would inside your office.

Fourth, features on your telemedicine application must have the ability to be turned on and off. Certain practices do not want all of the features that a robust telemedicine appointment can provide. For instance, many practices may not want patients to be able to text the practice or schedule new appointments. If that is the case, those features should be able to be turned "on" or "off" to satisfy your practice's needs. Additionally, branding and white labeling are critical for your practice to generate the trust necessary to compete well in the virtual healthcare world.

Finally, HD video and robust audio must be a part of every telemedicine service, especially for the surgical subspecialties. We rely so much on our ability to review and understand the appearance of wounds that HD video and audio quality is critically important. Any telemedicine software vendor that buffers their video for service strength at low bandwidth may be disturbing the clarity of the images that come across. This may be a liability threat to your organization.

Opportunities for Practice Growth

There are three main areas of practice opportunities that can be achieved with telemedicine. There is a clear hierarchy that is recommended as one becomes more advanced with your virtual medicine program. In the orthopedic space, postoperative visits are the low-hanging fruit and can provide significant return on investment.

Postoperative visits are especially beneficial in areas where radiographs are not necessary, such as arthroscopy and soft tissue procedures of the upper and lower extremity. In this scenario, one can utilize either asynchronous or synchronous telemedicine to achieve virtual visit goals. Asynchronous telemedicine can allow providers to be extremely efficient with postoperative visits, and this may allow providers to open up significant time on their schedules.

Established patient visits are next on the hierarchy of virtual visits and can be easily utilized in a variety of ways. Four main follow-up appointments are specific to telemedicine in orthopedics and include imaging follow-up, post-injection follow-up, preoperative surgical discussion, and chronic condition management. In orthopedics, imaging and testing follow-up is particularly easy to achieve with the screen sharing tools available with most telemedicine programs. These appointments can improve efficiency in the office, decrease overhead, and save patients' time.

Post-injection follow-up appointments are frequently performed by orthopedic surgeons and are generally done around 6 weeks. At these recheck appointments, providers will not provide another injection, but do want to inquire about patients' symptoms and their response to the injection. This is particularly useful with cortisone, platelet-rich plasma, and stem cells.

Preoperative surgical discussions, specifically for well-established patients, often require information transfer from the provider to the patient. Oftentimes, the surgeon has already examined the patient as well as reviewed the pertinent imaging. Many times, these surgical discussions may take place via a phone call; however, a live video conference discussing surgery can be reimbursed utilizing standard telemedicine billing codes.

It is also useful to monitor disease with telemedicine. Many orthopedic surgeons monitor diseases such as rotator cuff tears, meniscal tears, rheumatoid arthritis, and osteoarthritis at regular intervals. These visits are perfect for telemedicine follow-up but may require in-person visits because of injections, and so proper planning must occur. Lastly, the Centers for Medicare and Medicaid Services (CMS) is now reimbursing for chronic care management. Entrepreneurial orthopedic practices can monitor diseases such as arthritis and will be reimbursed for these appointments if they are done via telemedicine.

New patient visits are the highest level of orthopedic services that can be rendered via telemedicine. They provide the greatest opportunity for practice growth and can set your practice apart in your local and regional area. The new patient appointment can be achieved with the right infrastructure. Virtual urgent cares have sprung up across the country and represent a nice way to attract patients to your practice. Additional options for new patient consultation include a consultation kiosk present in your local internal medicine or urgent care office. Additionally, local employers with a high number of musculoskeletal injuries may appreciate having direct access to your practice through telemedicine.

Telemedicine allows us to modify the episodic care that we traditionally provide so that it now can span the continuum of their healthcare journey. We tend to evaluate patients at predetermined time intervals, although the patient's problem affects them every second of every day. With telemedicine, we can now interact with our patients in between those discrete episodes. Specifically, we can ensure that they are prepared and have appropriate expectations prior to an appointment and also debrief with them after an appointment to ensure that they understand the treatment plan and don't have any follow-up questions or concerns.

Some practices are considering direct-to-consumer telemedicine offerings through advertising on social media or through Google AdWords. This type of telemedicine offering has not proven to be successful yet in orthopedics, and questions remain whether the public will accept this model given that trust is so tightly tied to word of mouth in local communities.

Barriers to Telehealth Growth

Trust is the most significant barrier to orthopedic telehealth growth in the United States. Especially in the surgical subspecialties, trust can be difficult to demonstrate in an online environment. Thus, it is incredibly important to be able to utilize your local brand while providing telemedicine services in your community. An application that does not allow for you to market and brand will ultimately hurt your telemedicine business.

A significant hurdle among CEOs of orthopedic practices and hospitals when beginning their telemedicine program has been changing the practice patterns of physicians. Physicians are sometimes unable or unwilling to change their successful practice to accommodate telemedicine. Concerns exist over the potential loss of productivity and difficulty with technology. Many physicians experienced the transition to electronic health records and felt that the shift to telemedicine would cause similar efficiency losses. This has not been the case for telemedicine adopters, however. Multiple research articles point to the increased efficiency caused by telemedicine.

Other hurdles include Medicare telehealth laws which still require the patient to be in an appropriate rural service location. The potential service locations include a primary care physician's office, a rural health clinic, and other rural facilities. However, CMS is finalizing policies to bring innovative telehealth technologies to senior's homes, rather than requiring them to go to a healthcare facility [16]. Please refer to Chaps. 2 and 3 for a more detailed discussion of regulation, billing, and reimbursement.

Telemedicine laws are also not consistent on a state-to-state basis. This is why telehealth programs are confusing, and what may work in one state may not work in another. The most glaring example of this is the parity laws across the country. Certain states have parity laws that mandate that telemedicine visit reimbursement be equal to that of in-person visits. These laws are extremely beneficial, but even within parity states, the laws vary leaving decision-making with the insurers in some cases.

Nonetheless, cross-state licensure compacts are allowing for providers to more easily obtain medical licenses. If the practitioners in your practice see patients frequently from other states, it makes sense that they obtain these licenses since it does not require any additional paperwork. In the future, some consistency among states will bring much needed clarity so that telemedicine laws are the same among all of the states.

Expected Return on Investment

The expected return on investment for telemedicine is grounded in market research and has demonstrated a high rate of return for practices. In a report by Foley and Lardner's telehealth division, 50% of practices were following their return on investment from telemedicine. In those practices that were following their return on investment, over 50% saw a return on investment of 10% or more [17]. Other demonstrations of return on investment include studies performed in the orthopedic literature, like the study by Atanda et al. published in 2018 [8].

Examples of return on investment utilizing asynchronous telemedicine have shown extremely high rate of return on telemedicine. The diagrams/tables below provide a detailed analysis of how asynchronous telemedicine visits can decrease time and labor costs required to see patients compared to traditional, in-person visits. Specifically, these cost and time savings are most apparent with patients who are in the global (non-revenue generating) post-operative period.

Average Provider Productivity	
Variable	Amount
Participating Providers	28
Appointments/Provider/Day	40
Clinic Days/Week	2.5
Weeks/Year	44
Procedures/Year	440
Total Appointments	4400
Follow Up	1848
Post-Operative	1100
New	1452

Labor Cost Per Appointment		
Appt/Staff	Time	Cost
In-Office		
Mins/Post-Op MD/DO	10	$41.67
Mins/Post-Op MA	17	$5.67
Mins/Post-Op Staff	30	$8.00
Mins/ Follow Up MD/DO	10	$41.67
Mins/Follow Up MA	17	$5.67
Mins/Follow Up Staff	30	$8.00
Telemedicine		
Mins/Post-Op MD/DO	2	$8.33
Mins/Post-Op MA	5	$1.67
Mins/Post-Op Staff	5	$1.33
Mins/ Follow Up MD/DO	3	$12.50
Mins/ Follow Up MA	7	$2.33
Mins/ Follow Up Staff	7	$1.87

Eligible Post Operative Appts	
% Post-Operative Visits Eligible for Telemedicine	33%
Percent Patients Opt-In to Telemedicine	70%
Number of Post-Ops converted to telemedicine/year/provider	254

Eligible Routine Follow-Up Appts	
Percent of visits eligible for telemedicine	33%
Percent patients opt in to telemedicine	70%
Visits converted to telemedicine	427

Additional In-Office Visits (Time freed by Telemed)	
Telemedicine Appointments/Day	6.2
Mins saved/day- MD/DO	49.5
Mins required, New Patient Visit- MD/DO	13.0
Additional New Visits/Day	3.8

Assumptions

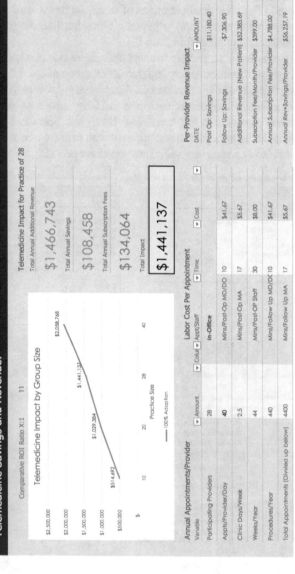

Telemedicine Savings and Revenue:

Comparative ROI Ratio X:1	11

Telemedicine Impact by Group Size

Telemedicine Impact for Practice of 28

Total Annual Additional Revenue

$1,466,743

Total Annual Savings

$108,458

Total Annual Subscription Fees

$134,064

Total Impact

$1,441,137

Annual Appointments/Provider

Variable	Amount
Participating Providers	28
Appts/Provider/Day	40
Clinic Days/Week	2.5
Weeks/Year	44
Procedures/Year	440
Total Appointments (Divvied up below)	4400

Labor Cost Per Appointment

Colum	Appt/Staff	Time	Cost
	In-Office		
	Mins/Post-Op MD/DO	10	$41.67
	Mins/Post-Op MA	17	$5.67
	Mins/Post-OP Staff	30	$8.00
	Mins/Follow Up MD/DC	10	$41.67
	Mins/Follow Up MA	17	$5.67

Per-Provider Revenue Impact

DATE	AMOUNT
Post Op: Savings	$11,180.40
Follow Up: Savings	-$7,306.90
Additional Revenue (New Patient)	$52,383.69
Subscription Fee/Month/Provider	$399.00
Annual Subscription Fees/Provider	$4,788.00
Annual Rev+Savings/Provider	$56,257.19

Six Steps of Telemedicine Development and Implementation

Brainstorming	In this phase, it is important to understand what your goals are with telemedicine inside your practice. Have internal meetings with all of your stakeholders to understand the potential applications for your practice.
Provider buy-in	After the decision has been made to consider telemedicine, it is important to gauge the temperature of your physicians. Some physicians are more likely to adopt new technology, and others are less likely to change. It is critical to have a physician champion or two to help create change within the practice.
Planning phase	During this phase, different technologies are explored, and hardware and software requirements are defined.
Provider/staff preparation	A telemedicine vendor is chosen, hardware and software are purchased, and a go-live date is established. Staff and provider training is performed. Workflows are planned.
Execution	Workflows are executed based on the planned implementation strategy. Any adjustments to the workflow can be made based on roadblocks and hurdles.
Process improvement	Every month, a meeting is held among the clinic staff to determine best practice for the telemedicine program and ensure patients and physicians are satisfied.

Please refer to the chart above to identify the six steps for tele-health development and implementation that are currently utilized at OrthoLive to improve successful implementation and rollout of a telemedicine program.

During the brainstorming phase, which should last about 2 weeks, but can last as long as 6 months, stakeholders from a specific practice will sit down and determine which types of tele-medicine visits are desired for the practice and what the time-frame for implementation will be and which providers will be the physician champions for the group.

Provider buy-in, the next stage, is a critically important phase that includes discussions at a board and group level to confirm the interest from the practitioners, so that the benefits of telemedicine can be established and the necessary steps explained. Without this important step, implementation can fail because physicians may be unwilling to change their practice accordingly. This is one of the most important steps in the development process for telemedicine.

Next is the planning phase. This can be a lengthy phase as it is critically important to thoroughly evaluate the different platforms available to determine which will be most effective for your practice. The telemedicine vendor may have an existing integration option for your electronic health record system which may make it more efficient for your staff. Below we have compiled a key list of features and "red flags." We encourage you to utilize this checklist as you identify a vendor that suits your practice goals. During this phase, you will see the different types of technology requirements demanded by each system. It is important for the system to meet your providers and patients where they most commonly are.

Important features:

1. Virtual waiting room
2. Notifications that patient is in the waiting room
3. Appointment reminders
4. Understanding when or if the patient has onboarded
5. Scheduling available by provider and patient

System "red flags":

1. System cannot white-label.
2. No appointment reminders.
3. No "waiting room."
4. No ring to notify patients who are outside the app that the provider is present.
5. Single web or mobile access for physicians.
6. No in-app messaging between patient and staff or provider and provider.
7. Provider can be messaged at any time by patient.
8. Inability to do video visits.
9. No text feature to download application.
10. No literature support for practice onboarding.

It is extremely important to choose a vendor who understands medical practice and created the application with the assistance of a medical professional. Without clinical input, many telemedicine applications may be cumbersome and not allow for easy use for the provider or the patient. For instance, a telehealth solution which only allows for web-based visits to occur essentially eliminates the ability for patients to be where they are most comfortable, which is on their phones. These simple and obvious issues are slowing telemedicine growth and creating frustration among providers.

In the preparation phase, several key timelines are established. First, it is important to determine a go-live date after you have signed your telemedicine software contract. Staff and provider preparation then begins and is usually led by your telemedicine vendor. Onsite or virtual demonstrations are performed to provide your staff with important information related to what, where, when, and how telemedicine is going to be performed at your institution. Workflows and processes are established during the preparation phase, so that all parties are involved in how telemedicine visits will be booked and run.

Finally, during the execution phase, telemedicine is implemented according to the planned protocols and processes. It is important that these processes be written down so that staff can understand how to go about scheduling and receiving telemedicine visits.

The last phase, process improvement, follows the execution phase. Meetings to improve process for telemedicine visits pay dividends in terms of increased efficiency and improved patient and provider reported satisfaction scores. No system is perfect on its first implementation, and the iterative process is one of the best ways to continue to improve everyone's satisfaction with their telemedicine experience.

Specific Use Cases for New Patient Telemedicine Development

Virtual Urgent Care: A virtual urgent care is an outstanding way to set your practice apart among the local and regional competitive marketplace. In best case scenarios, a brick-and-mortar urgent care has already been established by the practice. Utilizing the same staff, virtual appointments can be held which can be billed as a new patient appointment. Coding and billing, which is covered in another chapter, must include appropriate documentation.

The beauty of virtual appointments is that the practice can reach anyone, anywhere. Using targeted advertising and website traffic, new patients are likely to be able to get into the practice extremely quickly and easily. This also allows your practice to compete against the other direct-to-consumer telemedicine brands that are currently working with your potential patients.

Worker's Compensation: Virtual worker's compensation visits are already happening across the United States and represent a great opportunity for any practice that is currently working with employers. Employers want immediate access for their employees from their place of business, saving lost work time. There are a number of models that are already in place demonstrating how this can best be utilized. Please visit www.ortholive.com for more information on how worker's compensation programs can be implemented.

Sideline Coverage: Many orthopedic groups work with athletic trainers to cover football and basketball games at local high schools, colleges, universities, and professional sporting events. Telemedicine is extremely useful so that physicians can understand fully an injury sustained by an athlete. Especially in outlying areas, telemedicine can be extremely useful when an athletic trainer or physician is unavailable.

Outreach Clinics: In states where rural orthopedic coverage is poor, outreach clinics staffed by nurses or physician assistants and nurse practitioners can be a great way to see patients who may need orthopedic expertise but have poor access to care. In situations where orthopedic practitioners do not have a full schedule, these clinics can boost clinic visits and surgical volume.

Primary Care/Urgent Care Consultation: Availing the orthopedic practice to primary care and urgent care physicians is an extremely good way to generate new business and can improve relationships with these providers. Many urgent cares and primary care physicians are interested in providing immediate access to their consultants. Telemedicine provides a simple way to give immediate access to your orthopedic practice.

Triage Screening: Given the fee-for-service culture of our healthcare landscape, we are highly incentivized to see any patient that requests to enter our orthopedic ecosystem. As a result, we don't invariably know exactly what the patient needs or whether or not we can help them, until they are already standing in front of us. In the ambulatory setting, telemedicine offers the capability to visualize, evaluate, and obtain pertinent clinical information from patients *prior* to their appointment. This allows us to ensure that the patient in fact needs to be seen, that they are seeing the appropriate provider, and, most importantly, that they are being seen at the appropriate time.

Conclusions

Telemedicine is a new technology that supports both the physician and patient. When used correctly, it can provide significant customer satisfaction and can improve office efficiency. Using telemedicine locally can help orthopedic practices compete in their local community and can help prevent outside vendors from cherry-picking private pay patients who are marketing to them. Telemedicine implementation can be performed relatively easily inside a practice, but the abovementioned six steps should be followed to ensure success.

Works Cited

1. Houle D. The shift age: BookSurge; 2007.
2. (2019, June 12). Retrieved from Pew Research Center: https://www.pewresearch.org/internet/fact-sheet/mobile/.
3. Vearrrier L, Rosenberger K, Weber V. User of personal devices in healthcare: guidelines from a roundtable discussion. J Mob Technol Med. 2018;7(2):27–34.
4. Arise. 2019, February 20. Retrieved from https://www.arise.com/resources/blog/arise-customer-service-frustration-series-phone-hold-times

5. Open Market. 2016, May 5. Retrieved from https://www.openmarket. com/blog/millennials-prefer-text-over-talk/
6. Cole, N. 2017, April 25. Inc. Retrieved from inc.com: https://www.inc. com/nicolas-cole/the-power-of-live-chat-5-surprising-statistics-that-show-how-consumers-want-thei.html
7. Johnston KJ, Wen H, Joynt Maddox KE. Lack of access to specialists associated with mortality and preventable hospitalizations of rural medicare beneficiaries. Health Aff. 2019;38(12). epub ahead of print
8. Atanda A, Pelton M, Fabricant PD, Tucker A, Shah SA, Slamon N. Telemedicine utilisation in a paediatric sports medicine practice: decreased cost and wait times with increased satisfaction. J ISAKOS. 2018;3(2):94–7.
9. Schernhammer ES, Colditz GA. Suicide rates among physicians: a quantitative and gender assessment. Am J Psychiatry. Charleston; South Carolina. 2004;161(12):2295–302.
10. West CP, Dyrbye LN, Shanafelt TD. Physician burnout: contributors, consequences and solutions. J Intern Med. 2018;283(6):516–29.
11. Farmer, B. 2018, July 31. https://www.npr.org/sections/health-shots/2018/07/31/634217947/to-prevent-doctor-suicides-medical-industry-rethinks-how-doctors-work. Retrieved from NPR: http://www.npr.org
12. Arndt BG, Beasley JW, Watkinson MD, Temte JL, Tuan W-J, Sinsky CA, Gilchrist VJ. Tethered to the EHR: primary care physician workload assessment using EHR event log data and time-motion observations. Ann Fam Med. 2017;15(5):419–26.
13. (2018). Retrieved from Stanford University: https://med.stanford.edu/ content/dam/sm/ehr/documents/EHR-Poll-Presentation.pdf.
14. Howley MJ, Chou EY, Hansen N, Dalrymple PW. The long-term financial impact of electronic health record implementation. J Am Med Inform Assoc. 2015;22(2):443–52.
15. Mullen-Fortino M, Rising KL, Duckworth J, Gwynn V, Sites FD, Hollander JE. Presurgical assessment using telemedicine technology: impact on efficiency, effectiveness, and patient experience of care. Telemed J E Health. 2019;25(2):137–42.
16. CMS Press Releases. 2019, April 5. Retrieved from CMS.gov: https:// www.cms.gov/newsroom/press-releases/cms-finalizes-policies-bring-innovative-telehealth-benefit-medicare-advantage
17. Lacktman, N. 2017, November 8. Foley and Lardner. Retrieved from https://www.foley.com/files/uploads/2017-Telemedicine-Survey-Report-11-8-17.pdf

A Case Study in Telemedicine: Cerebral Palsy

M. Wade Shrader

Cerebral palsy (CP) is the most common cause of motor disability seen in childhood with an estimated annual incidence of approximately 2–4 per 1000 live births [1]. Historically, CP was caused by birth anoxia, but this has since changed with better obstetrical care. Prematurity is now a leading cause of CP as advanced neonatal resuscitation techniques have prolonged the lives of these children significantly.

The orthopedic surgeon becomes a cornerstone in the lives of many families who have children with cerebral palsy. These children often refer to their orthopedic surgeon as "their doctor," that is, the orthopedic surgeon is often the principal physician that cares for these children throughout their life span until they reach adulthood [2]. Because of the frequent clinical visits and surgical procedures, many families grow very close to their orthopedic surgeon and other members of the CP treatment team. This physical doctor-patient relationship is quite special, and therefore the use of telemedicine in the context of CP has not been widely accepted to date. However, these special-needs families have

M. W. Shrader (✉)
Department of Orthopedic Surgery, Nemours A.I. duPont Hospital for
Children, Wilmington, DE, USA
e-mail: wade.shrader@nemours.org

© Springer Nature Switzerland AG 2021
A. Atanda Jr., J. F. Lovejoy III (eds.), *Telemedicine in Orthopedic
Surgery and Sports Medicine*,
https://doi.org/10.1007/978-3-030-53879-8_9

many unique difficulties and challenges. Wheelchair-accessible transportation, parking, and coordination with multiple therapy services make the lives of these families quite complex. Therefore, having the option to have some of their healthcare delivered via telemedicine may be desirable for some of these families.

Postoperative wound checks for patients with CP may be very amenable to be conducted via telemedicine. Typical postoperative visits in CP patients usually are very quick but also have a very high cost to the patient in terms of time, expense, and travel, specifically for wheelchair patients. Telemedicine has been shown to demonstrate cost savings, excellent outcomes, and high patient satisfaction in orthopedic care using telemedicine for postoperative checks [3, 4].

Therapy services are also an attractive target for telemedicine in the cerebral palsy population. One randomized controlled trial demonstrated significant cost-effectiveness of a web-based multimodal therapy for unilateral cerebral palsy [5]. Patients who used this online training program demonstrated improved performance and satisfaction scales. Another randomized clinical trial used a telemedicine system to provide occupational therapy services and upper extremity exercises for children with hemiplegic cerebral palsy [6].

Gait analysis reviews for ambulatory children with cerebral palsy can very easily be done via telemedicine. At the point where it is felt that a turning point is reached in terms of the gait impairments affecting the child with CP, a complete three-dimensional computerized gait analysis is typically ordered. The timeframe between the review of the gait analysis with the family and initial clinical exam is frequently less than 8 weeks. As a result, the child's physical exam typically has not changed; therefore a repeat physical exam is not mandatory. Since many telemedicine platforms and applications have the ability to share screens, we are able to review the gait analysis with the family while they are home (Fig. 9.1). Using the split screen, we can review the videos, review the gait plots and data, and review and discuss our recommendations as if we were sitting in the same office together (Fig. 9.2). Reviewing the gait analysis in this manner saves time and cost by reducing the need for a formal in-person visit.

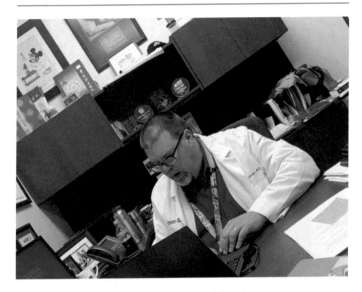

Fig. 9.1 Typical cerebral palsy gait review telehealth encounter

Although there is no specific data or evidence to support this utilization of telemedicine, our general impression is that families have a high satisfaction rate with this particular use case.

There are some limitations to utilizing telemedicine to care for cerebral patients that should be noted. We are unable to perform these gait analysis reviews in states where we are not licensed. Families must have some amount of tech literacy to be able to download and utilize the telemedicine software appropriately. Finally, given the personal and long-standing nature of the patient-provider relationships in CP patients, some families may prefer an in-person encounter depending on the clinical situation.

In conclusion, telemedicine may offer several opportunities for improved access to orthopedic care for children with cerebral palsy, especially in remote regions. Postoperative wound checks, gait analysis, and physical therapy visits are common examples of appropriate uses cases for CP patients. Telemedicine has the potential for improved convenience and satisfaction for the family to access those portions of care.

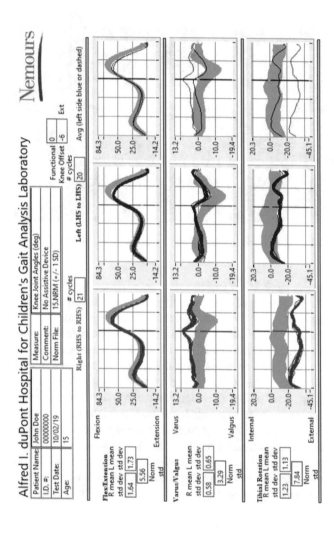

Fig. 9.2 Example of gait analysis kinematic data shared with the family through the telehealth encounter

References

1. Glader L, Plews-Ogan J, Argral R. Children with medical complexity: creating a framework for care based on the international classification of functioning, disability and health. Dev Med Child Neurol. 2016;58:1116–23.
2. Miller F, editor. Cerebral palsy. New York: Springer; 2006.
3. Sharareh B, Scharzakopf R. Effectiveness of telemedical applications in postoperative follow-up after total joint arthroplasty. J Arthroplast. 2014;29(5):918–22.
4. Atanda A, Pelton M, Fabricant PD, Tucker A, Shah SA, Slamon N. Telemedicine in a pediatric sports medicine practice: decreased cost and wait times and increased satisfaction. JISAKOS. 2018;0:1–4. https://doi.org/10.1136/jisakos-2017-000176.
5. Comans T, Mihala G, Sakewski L, Boyd RN, Scuffham P. The cost-effectiveness of a web-based multi-modal therapy for unilateral cerebral palsy: the Mitii randomized controlled trial. Dev Med Child Neurol. 2017;59(7):756–61.
6. Sgandurra G, Cecchi F, Beani E, Mannari I, Maselli M, Falotico FP, Inguaggiato E, Perazza S, Sicola E, Feys H, Klingels K, Ferrari A, Dario P, Boyd RN, Cioni G. Tele-UPCAT: study protocol of a randomized controlled trial of a home-based Tele-monitored upper limb children action observation training for participants with unilateral cerebral palsy. BMJ Open. 2018;8(5):e017819.

10 Provider-to-Provider Telemedicine Consultation

Sean Tackett and Emmanuel Opati

Most patients with acute and chronic musculoskeletal problems initially present to another provider prior to presentation to the orthopedic provider. Orthopedic surgeons, like many subspecialists, often have barriers around them that preclude patients from seeing them as the initial point of contact. These include geography, in the case of rural patients, or availability, in the case of when the specialist is occupied in the operating room or clinic. Limited access to specialists is especially acute in low- and middle-income countries, which will be discussed in Chap. 17 "International Clinical and Educational Initiatives." As a result, emergency rooms, urgent care centers, and primary care offices are often the first clinical touchpoint for these patients as these entities are often accessible, available, known to them, and in their home communities. These initial touchpoints are very equipped at providing pain control, temporizing treatment, and offering preliminary education about the patient's problem. However, the true essence of what the

S. Tackett
Johns Hopkins Bayview Medical Center, Baltimore, MD, USA
e-mail: stacket1@jhmi.edu

E. Opati (✉)
XpertCare Inc., Baltimore, MD, USA
e-mail: emmanuelopati@xpertcare.online

A. Atanda Jr., J. F. Lovejoy III (eds.), *Telemedicine in Orthopedic Surgery and Sports Medicine*,
https://doi.org/10.1007/978-3-030-53879-8_10

patient needs is clinical guidance, advice, recommendations, and a formal treatment plan. Questions most patients have include the following: When can I go back to school/work? When can I put weight on my leg? Do I need to sleep in the brace you provided? When will I be able to play sports again? How much pain should I expect? The initial providers don't always provide precise answers to these questions, whether it be for lack of knowledge, lack of time, or fear of liability. Moreover, the idea of when, if, and how the patient should follow up with an orthopedic specialist is not always clear during these initial visits. As a result, patients may leave these visits somewhat dissatisfied and confused about their problem. In addition, the patients may wind up following up at an inappropriate time with the specialist. Ultimately, they will likely need to follow up with an orthopedist to be evaluated and have their questions answered. Unfortunately, the timing at which they get a follow-up appointment can be variable, and not having a definitive treatment plan during that time interval can be frustrating and a large source of anxiety and stress for the patients. From the orthopedist's perspective, it may be frustrating and wasteful to have to evaluate patients that may have been initially given inappropriate expectations of how the patient may be treated. Moreover, a subset of the patients that are referred to you in this manner may not need to see you at all and could've been managed by their primary care provider. Although these nonessential visits generate revenue, they also take up clinic slots from patients that may need surgery or have more complex problems.

Telehealth technology offers a potential solution to streamline this process as it can allow for the movement of knowledge, data, and information as opposed to the movement of patients. This can facilitate more rapid and efficient access to specialist expertise, overcoming geographic, temporal, and knowledge barriers. As an orthopedist, most of your diagnostic power lies in the imaging (i.e., X-rays, CT scans, and MRIs) that is obtained on your patient. By creating infrastructures, reliable methods, and workflows to move knowledge and imaging studies efficiently and systematically, one has the ability to streamline the treatment and triage process of orthopedic patients as they begin the journey of dealing with their injury or condition.

Generally, provider-to-provider options can be grouped into synchronous and asynchronous consultations. Synchronous consultations refer to transfer of health-related data and information in real time between two providers to deliver medical expertise. Asynchronous consults do not involve real-time interactions but rather capture data and information (pictures, video, text, audio) at one site and subsequently transmit this data and information to another site for interpretation by a healthcare professional. Here we'll define and provide examples of common synchronous and asynchronous methods. Note that asynchronous and synchronous methods can be complementary (e.g., asynchronous exchange can lead to synchronous discussion). Also note that while we focus on provider-to-provider consultations in this chapter, often a specialist provider will interact with both the consulting provider and patient at the same time.

The most important factors when selecting a consultation modality are how urgent the nature of the request is and the level of complexity of the clinical scenario. Unpredictable and urgent requests (such as those originating from ICUs or emergency departments) have different technical and staffing requirements than more predictable and less urgent requests (such as those originating from outpatient settings) and typically require synchronous provider interactions. Non-urgent requests may be best suited to asynchronous methods. Sometimes very complex cases that require one or more subspecialist may require more time to find the appropriate provider(s) to render an opinion.

Synchronous Examples: On-Demand/Urgent Consultations

Patients suffering injuries that require orthopedic surgical evaluation often first present to an urgent care center or emergency department. Emergency department or urgent care center providers then must refer patients to hospitals for orthopedic surgical evaluation. Patients can wait long hours in an emergency department for an orthopedic surgeon to arrive in their room after they have completed clinic, finished operating, and/or traveled from home or another hospital they were covering. By leveraging tele-health technologies, one can provide more rapid access to care, minimize resource utilization, and avoid unnecessary delays.

Pure provider-provider synchronous on-demand/urgent consultations are generally rare. Telestroke is one example [1], where in some cases providers can render an emergent opinion by relying on the neurologic exam of another provider conducted over telephone [2]. However, most tele-orthopedics requires visual evaluation of a patient, and we were unable to find published instances of urgent tele-orthopedic models that did not include patients. It's like that urgent provider-to-provider tele-orthopedic options require inclusion of a patient in the clinical evaluation.

When an on-demand/urgent consultation is required, certain practical limitations must be considered. These consultations often require rapid access to clinical data and providers. Using the same EHR is highly advantageous if possible. If providers do not have access to the same EHR, then other (HIPAA-secure) options must be used to share data, images, text, and other clinical information. Video technologies can be useful for emergency providers to demonstrate physical exam findings. If video is not available and imaging is insufficient, the surgeons may be able to address the scenario by phone if they can trust the provider's examination. This may be possible in programs where emergency providers have received training or with graduate medical trainees. Ideally surgeons should document their opinions themselves; this is straightforward when EHRs are shared but requires some method of record sharing otherwise.

On-demand case example no. 1

> Mr. Jones suffers an ankle injury and is taken to a local urgent care. X-rays show an ankle fracture that the provider thinks might require surgery. The provider wants an orthopedic surgery evaluation, so he calls a hotline and speaks with an orthopedic surgeon who views the images and observes the urgent care provider performing a physical exam. The surgeon requests specific exam maneuvers and coaches the provider through them. He recommends follow-up in clinic. Mr. Jones is splinted, prescribed pain medication, and discharged home with instructions to follow up in the outpatient clinic later in the week.

On-demand case example no. 2

Ms. Smith is in a medical ICU in a rural location recovering from sepsis. She is participating in physical therapy while on a ventilator when she falls and sustains a knee injury. X-rays show a significantly displaced patella fracture. No orthopedic surgeons are available within a 100 mile radius. A surgeon is given remote access, reviews the X-rays, and evaluates the patient remotely with the ICU provider present. The surgeon recommends urgent operative fixation, and the patient is subsequently transferred to a tertiary care center for definitive management.

Asynchronous Examples: eConsults and Remote Medical Second Opinions

Musculoskeletal complaints are very common in the outpatient primary care setting. Obtaining real-time orthopedic expertise at this initial point of contact is rarely possible. Traditional workflows require a subsequent orthopedic specialist visit which inevitably requires more time off from work/school, can present delays in care, may leave providers uncertain about the plan of care, and leave patients confused, anxious, and in pain. Various forms of eConsultations can expedite care and streamline this process by creating an infrastructure to transfer knowledge, guidance, and advice from the specialist to the primary provider in a more rapid manner.

For example, many EHRs now offer and facilitate **eConsult** requests, and some institutions have developed their own eConsult platforms. PCPs can send the request asynchronously to a specialist, who can then review the pertinent clinical information and document their opinion. A recent review documented that EHR-based eConsults have been shown to decrease wait times for specialists, are acceptable, can increase provider satisfaction, and can reduce cost [3], and a statewide evaluation that included orthopedic surgeons similarly showed reduced face-to-face consults and cost [4]. In addition to healthcare systems, there are private vendors that have developed virtual networks of specialists and compliant eConsult platforms where PCPs can send the request asynchronously with pertinent clinical information for the specialists to render their opinions.

eConsult case example

> Mr. Wilson sees his PCP after hurting his back. The PCP performs an exam and obtains the appropriate X-rays but is uncertain whether or not an MRI is warranted. When he documents his note, he sends an eConsult request to an orthopedic surgeon for advice about the utility of an MRI. The surgeon reviews the pertinent clinical information and imaging. The surgeon suggests physical therapy, NSAIDs, and activity modification and to hold off on the MRI for now. The PCP then relays this message to Mr. Wilson and begins the treatment plan.

Even after patients have seen a specialist, they may still want a second opinion from a subsequent specialist. In addition, some specialists may want input from a more-experienced physician to help treat a specific clinical problem. There are many private vendors that offer **remote medical second-opinion** services. Most of these vendors cater to patients who would like their images, laboratory data, and other medical records remotely reviewed by a specialist. This has the added benefit of saving time, energy, and money for the patient if the remote opinion can prevent unnecessary travel. The turnaround time for opinion and review to be completed is typically more flexible and can range from a couple of days to a couple of weeks. While many large, self-insured employers pay for remote medical second opinions for their employees, insurance companies often do not, and patients must bear the cost. Given the fact that orthopedic decision-making is primarily based on imaging, there may be many opportunities for second opinions to be utilized in orthopedic practices. One study of a remote medical second-opinion program in the United States found that orthopedic surgery was the most frequently requested among 34 specialties. Their second opinions resulted in changes in diagnosis in 14% and changes in treatment plans in 35% of cases [5].

Remote medical second-opinion case example

> Ms. Walker sees a surgeon in clinic who recommends surgery for ongoing shoulder pain. She is not sure if she needs the surgery, so she wants an opinion from another surgeon. She acquires her records and imaging and sends them to a commercial vendor who

routes them to a shoulder specialist. Two weeks later, she receives the specialist's written opinion stating that surgery is also recommended. Ms. Walker returns to the original surgeon for preoperative planning.

Asynchronous and Synchronous: eBoard

Complex cases may require input from multiple specialists and often involve asynchronous information-sharing and synchronous discussions among providers. For example, oncologic problems often require collaboration between surgeons, oncologists, pathologists, and radiation oncologists. Teleoncology can support patients at all stages of their cancer care [6]. Tumor boards are common in cancer care, and telehealth modalities can allow providers to participate in virtual tumor boards from remote settings [7]. As diagnostics become more sophisticated, computational methods may play a bigger role in supporting providers working in a multidisciplinary team [8].

Self-Service

In some rare instances, algorithms can be developed and placed online so that provider, or their patients, can input a limited set of variables to determine whether surgery is needed or not. This is most useful when surgical expertise is very specialized and a patient would almost certainly be required to travel to receive their care.

Challenges to Provider-to-Provider Consultations

Reimbursement: Uncertainty about reimbursement remains one of the biggest barriers to telemedicine generally. Although about 42 states have some form of telehealth statue for commercial payers, only 10 states mandate payment parity, meaning that telemedicine services must have similar reimbursement rates as in-person services [9].

Providers are also not yet comfortable with the technology required to set up and run a provider-to-provider consultation service. Technology can be overwhelming and often explained by vendors who have limited experience with its practical application and integration in an orthopedic practice. There are some off-the-shelf telemedicine platforms that are compliant with federal and state regulations and also easy to set up and run. Another technical challenge is appropriate and meaningful integration in the clinic workflow to optimize both clinical and financial outcomes.

The legal framework is improving as the federal government, states, providers, and patients push for more access to high-quality care. The Department of Veteran Affairs (VA) has been leading in piloting and instituting telemedicine services across various VA-run hospitals.

Also note that reimbursement rules are constantly changing, although increasingly national payors are reimbursing for synchronous and asynchronous telehealth methods [10]. There are also a variety of employers who pay for remote medical second opinions.

- Clinic workflow integration
- HIPAA-compliant platform/interoperability
- Providers on both ends comfortable with technology
- Legal and ethical framework for the licensure/medical malpractice

References

1. Wechsler LR, Demaerschalk BM, Schwamm LH, Adeoye OM, Audebert HJ, Fanale CV, Rosamond WD. Telemedicine quality and outcomes in stroke: a scientific statement for healthcare professionals from the American Heart Association/American Stroke Association. Stroke. 2017;48(1):e3–e25.
2. Majersik JJ, Meurer WJ, Frederiksen SA, Sandretto AM, Xu Z, Goldman EB, Scott PA. Observational study of telephone consults by stroke experts supporting community tissue plasminogen activator delivery. Acad Emerg Med. 2012;19(9):E1027–34.

3. Liddy C, Moroz I, Mihan A, Nawar N, Keely E. A systematic review of asynchronous, provider-to-provider, electronic consultation services to improve access to specialty care available worldwide. Telemed J E Health. 2019;25(3):184–98.
4. Anderson D, Villagra VG, Coman E, Ahmed T, Porto A, Jepeal N, Teevan B. Reduced cost of specialty care using electronic consultations for Medicaid patients. Health Aff. 2018;37(12):2031–6.
5. Meyer AN, Singh H, Graber ML. Evaluation of outcomes from a national patient-initiated second-opinion program. Am J Med. 2015;128(10):1138–e25.
6. Shalowitz DI, Smith AG, Bell MC, Gibb RK. Teleoncology for gynecologic cancers. Gynecol Oncol. 2015;139(1):172–7.
7. Marshall CL, Petersen NJ, Naik AD, Velde NV, Artinyan A, Albo D, Anaya DA. Implementation of a regional virtual tumor board: a prospective study evaluating feasibility and provider acceptance. Telemed J E Health. 2014;20(8):705–11.
8. Pishvaian MJ, Blais EM, Bender RJ, Rao S, Boca SM, Chung V, Moore KN. A virtual molecular tumor board to improve efficiency and scalability of delivering precision oncology to physicians and their patients. JAMIA Open. 2019;2(4):505–15.
9. Lacktman MN, Acosta NJ, Levine JS. 50 state survey of telehealth commercial payer statues. Folley.com; 2019
10. ATA (2019). Telehealth Benefits (n.d.). Retrieved from https://www.americantelemed.org/resource/why-telemedicine/.

Direct-to-Consumer Telemedicine

11

Patricia Solo-Josephson,
Cynthia M. Zettler-Greeley,
and Joanne Murren-Boezem

Direct-to-Consumer Telemedicine

Telemedicine is a term coined in the 1970s, which means "healing at a distance." In direct-to-consumer (DTC) telemedicine, the consumer (patient) requests a visit and connects to a healthcare provider using a computer or mobile device from the comfort of their home, school, or work. Bringing the provider to the patient, albeit virtually, recalls the age-old house calls, with a modern technological twist. DTC telemedicine platforms typically operate 24 hours a day, 7 days a week, making around-the-clock access to a healthcare provider and convenience to the patient two of its paramount features. The impact is less (or no) travel time, reduced exposure to other ill patients, and the potential for rapid diagnosis and treatment. Consequently, a common characteristic of many DTC programs is high patient satisfaction [1, 2].

P. Solo-Josephson (✉) · C. M. Zettler-Greeley · J. Murren-Boezem
Nemours Children's Health System, Center for Health Delivery
Innovation, Orlando, FL, USA
e-mail: Patricia.solojosephson@nemours.org;
Cynthia.zettlergreeley@nemours.org;
Joanne.murrenboezem@nemours.org

© Springer Nature Switzerland AG 2021
A. Atanda Jr., J. F. Lovejoy III (eds.), *Telemedicine in Orthopedic Surgery and Sports Medicine*,
https://doi.org/10.1007/978-3-030-53879-8_11

As with other telemedicine models, DTC health information transmission can take one of several forms. *Synchronous* care allows providers to deliver medical expertise to patients via real-time videoconferencing, email, or texting. Videoconferencing typically occurs through a HIPAA-compliant telemedicine platform, which allows for face-to-face communication between a patient and provider [2]. Patients initiate contact with a provider on the platform and, once connected, can share their health concerns directly, receiving immediate feedback.

Asynchronous telemedicine, also known as "store-and-forward," is utilized when health information is collected and later sent to a healthcare provider, such as when a patient transmits his/her medical history, biosensor readings, or images to a specialist for diagnostic review and treatment expertise. Patient-initiated, asynchronous telemedicine may simply involve email communication with a provider or may occur via store-and-forward telemedicine platforms, mobile health ("m-health") applications, software, or websites [3, 4]. Patients and providers can communicate at their convenience, as they are not connected in real time.

Remote patient monitoring (RPM) involves continuous evaluation of a patient's clinical status, whether through direct video monitoring of the patient or via review of tests and images collected remotely. Patients are given a remote device by their healthcare provider that monitors the patient's vital signs, oxygen levels, blood sugar, heart rate, weight, and other health data, sending it directly to the physician [5]. Although evidence is mixed, some studies suggest RPM correlates with reduced length of stay in hospital and lower hospital readmission rates [6].

Whereas standard telemedicine encounters typically involve examination of ailments that can be diagnosed through audiovisual means, the extent of chief complaints that can be diagnosed virtually is expanded by the use of home peripheral devices, which connect to smartphones, tablets, or computers. Although such home exam kits are not yet commonplace, patients utilizing these devices enable remote physicians to auscultate heart and lung sounds, detect fevers, and diagnose high blood pressure, ear infections, and numerous skin ailments, via synchronous or asynchronous transmissions [7].

Common origins of visit access include the patient's home, work, or school, although DTC telemedicine can operate anywhere a patient has a mobile device or computer and a reliable Internet connection. Visits in the school setting are relatively more complex than in other settings. Whereas most urgent care telemedicine visits are facilitated by adult patients themselves, school visits involving child patients typically are facilitated by a MA or the school nurse [8]. Privacy and confidentiality of health information, as obtained by and transmitted in schools, are governed by HIPAA as well as FERPA (Family Educational Rights and Privacy Act) [8]. The American Telemedicine Association (ATA) guidelines, also endorsed by the American Academy of Pediatrics (AAP), state that the child's primary care pediatrician should be informed of the visit, as the telemedicine encounter is seen as a "complement" to the patient-centered medical home [9]. In addition, enrollment forms, completed prior to the child's initial visit, should include a signed parental consent and describe parental involvement in visits [8]. Verbal consent should be attempted from the child at the time of visit, and the child's parent should be invited to participate in the encounter, either in person or virtually [8]. School-based telemedicine will be discussed in a thorough detail in a subsequent chapter.

Patient-initiated, DTC telemedicine delivers acute primary care services that often are provided by third-party companies [10] and commonly serves as a substitute for urgent care visits [1]. Procedurally, in a synchronous DTC telemedicine visit, the patient first creates an online account with the desired platform and enters demographic, pharmacy, and payment information. The patient appears in a virtual waiting room where a provider is notified and accepts the connection through a secure portal. After the medical history and physical exam are completed, the provider reviews the treatment plan with the patient, and prescriptions are sent electronically, if deemed necessary. The after-visit summary is forwarded to the patient's email with a copy kept securely on the platform for future use by the patient.

Benefits of DTC Telemedicine

DTC telemedicine appeals to healthcare consumers because it is faster, more convenient, and more mobile than an office visit. The advantage of providing timely and convenient services, particularly to remote locations and after normal business hours, drives its use among consumers today. According to a Cisco global survey, 76% of patients prioritize access to care over human contact with a provider [11]. Likewise, 70% of patients stated they were comfortable communicating with their healthcare providers via text, email, or video, in lieu of seeing them in person [11]. In today's healthcare market, consumerism is one of the main forces behind the surge in DTC utilization.

DTC telemedicine offers prompt and efficient care when an acute illness affects a family. In the United States, children younger than 15 years of age make up an estimated 70 million office visits annually for acute problems [12]. As 40% of work-related absences are due to a young child's illness [13, 14], DTC telemedicine provides a convenient alternative to an in-person visit when obtaining clearance for sending children back to school and parents back to work [15]. DTC telemedicine also gives families an opportunity to seek more economical care in lieu of more costly options. Of families using a DTC platform, 76% reported they would have pursued an urgent care center, emergency room (ER), or retail clinic in the absence of telemedicine [2]. Notably, non-urgent ER visits are about seven times more costly than DTC telemedicine [15]. Appropriate redirection from more costly services may offer potential cost savings, but further research is needed to fully understand the impact of DTC telemedicine on utilization and cost.

By overcoming geographic barriers, DTC telemedicine improves access for patients in remote communities. As noted by the National Rural Health Association, the patient-to-primary care physician ratio in rural areas is 39.8 physicians per 100,000 people, compared to 53.3 physicians per 100,000 in urban areas [16]. By eliminating inconvenient and costly travel, DTC telemedicine bridges the gap and allows rural families more equitable access to care [17]. Through a decrease in automobile travel and fuel consumption, DTC telemedicine also benefits the environment. A large-scale study at UC Davis demonstrated how a university outpatient consultation telemedicine program resulted in a total travel distance savings of 5,345,602 miles [18]. These savings resulted in a travel-related emission reduction of 1969 metric tons of carbon dioxide, 50 metric tons of carbon monoxide, 3.7 metric tons of nitrogen oxides, and 5.5 metric tons of volatile organic compounds and an overall decrease in fuel consumption [18]. Hence, DTC telemedicine overcomes geographic barriers and decreases travel time and distance while reducing travel-related emissions, thus contributing to a positive impact on the environment.

Of all the benefits of DTC telemedicine, perhaps none are so great as their value realized during crises as diverse as the COVID-19 pandemic of 2020 and extreme weather events [19, 20, 21]. During a pandemic, telemedicine preserves essential patient access to care while maintaining the integrity of "shelter in place" orders, thus mitigating infection exposure among healthcare workers and reducing illness transmission [19]. Likewise, when in-person visits are difficult or impossible to attend due to an impending natural disaster, DTC platforms offer seamless transitions from routine operations to disaster readiness, as physicians can be enlisted quickly from large provider networks to serve an influx of patients [21]. During Hurricane Irma in September 2017, a pediatric DTC telemedicine platform remained operational while successfully meeting increased patient demand, which peaked the day before the storm [21]. Findings suggested that DTC telemedicine may provide significant support during all three phases of emergency relief: pre-, mid-, and post-disaster. Additional research on streamlining and incorporating DTC telemedicine platforms into emergency disaster relief programs should be considered.

Finally, DTC telemedicine offers patients access to specialty care, such as dermatology and mental health. DTC teledermatology now offers 22 services in the United States [22], expanding reasonably affordable access to care in states having a short supply of board-certified dermatologists [22, 23]. Likewise, remotely delivered, behavioral health interventions as administered by licensed clinical social workers and behavioral coaches are shown to reduce overall resource utilization among enrolled cardiac patients, including reductions in hospital admission rates, while recognizing cost savings [24]. Whether DTC telemedicine is used to offload patients, as in an urgent care model, or is utilized in the management of specific medical conditions, DTC telemedicine brings value to individual consumers and to specialty groups in the healthcare industry.

Barriers to DTC Telemedicine Adoption

Driven by convenience, patient-initiated telemedicine is rapidly growing. Globally, the DTC services market is expected to reach 470 mil USD by 2025, with a compound annual growth rate (CAGR) of 5.6% over each of the next 5 years [25]. Despite its considerable growth, telemedicine remains underutilized as a form of healthcare, currently accounting for 6–11% of all patient encounters [26]. Numerous barriers constrain more widespread adoption. These barriers, largely, though not exclusively endemic to DTC telemedicine, can be classified into three ways: patient barriers, provider barriers, and industry barriers.

Patient Barriers Broadband Internet technology and pervasive use of smartphones and tablets with sophisticated cameras have powered the evolution of DTC telemedicine, the technological boon underpinning "anytime, anywhere" healthcare. As noted, much of the success of DTC telemedicine has been propelled by consumer demand for access to timely convenient healthcare, which largely is driven by the technologically savvy millennial generation. In 2019, over 13% of adults aged 18–24 years utilized telemedicine; yet only 5.3% of patients over 65 did so [26]. Lack of awareness and/or concern over care coordination may explain the relatively lower uptake among senior patients, who are more likely to believe that the quality of care received via telemedicine is inferior to an in-person visit [26]. Yet, studies support strong quality of care with DTC telemedicine, showing findings consistent with treatment received in urgent care and emergency departments [27]. Patient adoption is constrained by knowledge of telemedicine availability; over 80% of patients are unaware that their primary care physician (PCP) offers the service [26]. Likewise, access to necessary technology may hinder DTC telemedicine use among many potential patients and is of particular concern for patients in rural communities, who may not have sufficient home Internet speeds for supporting videoconferencing visits [28]. As a vulnerable group, patients residing in rural communities experience higher rates of chronic conditions and poorer health outcomes than patients in urban environments [29]. Such patients stand to benefit the most from remote healthcare, as lengthy commutes to urgent care facilities or emergency departments can delay critical or life-saving treatment. Whereas encrypted transmission of patient data is the norm, technology fears, including the possibility of data breaches during the transmission of protected health information via the Internet, may discourage potential users [30]. Costs for a DTC telemedicine visit vary, and patients may be reluctant to use the service before understanding any applicable insurance reimbursements. Nevertheless, even out-of-pocket DTC visits are a reasonably priced healthcare option for many patients, with an average cost of about 40–60 USD for a 15-minute visit with a provider.

Use of DTC often means patients are obtaining care outside of the medical home, which may fragment care and inspire quality concerns. Storage of patient data for privately run platforms operated outside of a patient's home healthcare system may not be affiliated with the patient's existing electronic health record (EHR). Because of the lack of a preexisting patient-provider relationship, patients may question the provider's qualifications or knowledge of their condition. Moreover, non-use of peripheral devices limits what complaints are appropriate for virtual examination, and patients may be unaware how or whether they might benefit from their use. Finally, where an examination culminates with a prescription for follow-up testing – a culture, blood draw, or others – research indicates that many telemedicine patients are unlikely to follow through on the recommendation [31].

Provider Barriers Barriers to provider adoption of DTC include legal and regulatory requirements that govern telemedicine as a whole. Rapidly evolving inter- and intrastate policies concerning reimbursement, liability, and licensure present a challenge to navigate [32]. Licensure requirements limit the extent to which a provider can extend his or her reach to patients around the country. Indeed, access to care for populations in underserved communities may be constrained by federal requirements for physicians to obtain medical licensure in every state in which his or her patients reside [33]. To ease this restriction, an Interstate Medical Licensure Compact (IMLC) was launched in 2017, expediting licensure for physicians who hold a medical license in a participating state and wish to practice medicine in additional states belonging to the Compact. Currently, 24 states and 1 US territory participate in the Compact; another 5 states and the District of Columbia have sought permission to join [34].

Providers, like their patients, may be apprehensive about utilizing digital technology for a medical examination. Concerns over accuracy and reliability of equipment or questions pertaining to its use may limit adoption, as well as questions about how its implementation might be integrated into the existing workflow [35, 36]. Moreover, a provider on a DTC platform typically is restricted to audiovisual examination as patients make contact via a tablet or smartphone as peripheral device use remains under-represented. DTC quality assurance has been questioned, as patient satisfaction ratings have been linked to unnecessary antibiotic prescription dispensing for patients with upper respiratory infections [1]. In specialties that rely heavily on physical examination and imaging studies, such as orthopedic surgery, many providers are skeptical of how well they can evaluate a patient through DTC models. However, as seen in previous chapters, there are many ways that virtually examine patients with musculoskeletal complaints. Further, DTC evaluation in orthopedics should be thought more as a triage screening tool as opposed to a tool used for definitive diagnosis and treatment.

Industry Barriers There is some evidence that greater access to care leads to increased use of healthcare resources [37]. Although telemedicine use may represent a lower one-to-one cost ratio with emergency department visits, urgent care, or in-person office visits, satisfaction surveys conducted with telemedicine users demonstrate that a small percentage of patients would have "done nothing" if they had not had access to telemedicine. Such users effectively represent an increase in healthcare utilization [37]. A second concern specific to DTC telemedicine is the extent to which its use contributes to the fragmentation of healthcare [38]. Fragmentation – the extent to which a patient's healthcare is delivered by multiple providers having little communication with one another and relatively limited knowledge of the patient's medical history – is a quality concern that is endemic to "transactional medicine." Whereas DTC platforms that are incorporated within health systems often have mechanisms in place to help combat this issue – for instance, sending the after-visit summary to the patient's PCP following a telemedicine visit – fragmentation may occur if the patients choose not to disclose their primary care provider's contact information or if a provider on a commercial platform doesn't request the information during the visit. Moreover, even *within* health systems that offer telemedicine, EHR integration with DTC platforms remains a challenge: A 2018 survey of healthcare professionals revealed that only 25.8% of health systems integrated their on-demand telemedicine into the EHR [39].

Overcoming Barriers Although the list of barriers to DTC adoption and utilization is extensive, many can be overcome with patient and provider education. Patient education from providers and other trusted industry experts who champion the technology should center on appropriate uses of DTC telemedicine to promote suitable uses and minimize its potential for overuse, serving to complement, rather than fragment, continuity of care. Likewise, physician education by experienced platform technicians who assuage privacy concerns, demonstrate equipment use, and support integration into workflows may assist in promoting DTC adoption. In addition, legislative victories, motivated by the consumer demand for access to high-quality, affordable, convenient healthcare, continue to ease restrictions on regulatory requirements. Lastly, a growing number of healthcare systems now include DTC telemedicine as a care option for their patients – increasing convenience and improving access, especially after hours – while retaining quality and maintaining the integrity of the medical home [2].

Future Directions

In spite of numerous barriers, the future of telemedicine is bright. Telemedicine is poised to play a major role as healthcare shifts into a value-based model, increasing access to care to improve patient health outcomes at lower cost. Economists who support the value of the healthcare technology are proposing state licensure mandate alternatives to policymakers, such as the proposal for one national license [40]. Such legislative actions would serve to increase telemedicine adoption and would be especially impactful for patient-initiated DTC. US infrastructure improvements are bringing broadband technology to rural areas, offering support for increased DTC access among a larger population of potential users [41]. Further expansion of the technology into schools, nursing homes, cruise ships, and other domains where people can benefit from immediate and convenient access to healthcare will capture the unique value of DTC. Use of telehealth peripheral devices, now available at some technology retailers, is expected to grow. Importantly, patient satisfaction with telemedicine remains high. The continued proliferation of satisfied patients and provider ambassadors ensures that DTC telemedicine will re-shape current models of primary and urgent care as the expectation of immediate access to quality healthcare for patients and families continues to rise.

References

1. Martinez KA, Rood M, Jhangiani N, et al. Patterns of use and correlates of patient satisfaction with a large nationwide direct to consumer telemedicine service. J Gen Intern Med. 2018;33(10):1768–73. https://doi.org/10.1007/s11606-018-4621-5.
2. Vyas S, Murren-Boezem J, Solo-Josephson P. Analysis of a pediatric telemedicine program. Telemed J E Health. 2018;24(12):993–7.

3. Lau C, Churchill RS, Kim J, et al. Asynchronous, web-based, patient-centered, home telemedicine system. IEEE Trans Biomed Eng. 2002;49(12):1452–62.
4. Website: mHealthIntelligence.com. Asynchronous telehealth gives providers an alternative to DTC video. Accessed at https://mhealthintelligence.com/news/asynchronous-telehealth-gives-providers-an-alternative-to-dtc-video
5. Center for Connected Health Policy. Remote patient monitoring (RPM). Accessed at https://www.cchpca.org/about/about-telehealth/remote-patient-monitoring-rpm
6. Freitag TB, Taylor G, Wick L, et al. Novel remote patient monitoring system improves key outcomes. J Card Fail. 2019;25(8):S104.
7. McDaniel NL, Novicoff W, Gunnell B, et al. Comparison of a novel handheld telehealth device with stand-alone examination tools in a clinic setting. Telemed J E Health. 2019;25(12):1225–30.
8. McSwain SD, Burke BL, Dharmar M, et al. American telemedicine association operating procedures for pediatric Telehealth. Telemed J E Health. 2017;23(9):699–706.
9. Gough F, Budhrani S, Cohn E, et al. ATA practice guidelines for live, on-demand primary and urgent care. Telemed J E Health. 2015;21(3):233–41.
10. Yu J, Mink PJ, Huckfeldt PJ, et al. Population-level estimates of telemedicine service provision using an all-payer claims database. Health Aff. 2018;37:1931–9.
11. Cisco. Survey: 76% of patients would choose telehealth over human contact. Available at http://hitconsultant.net/2013/03/08/survey-patients-would-choose-telehealth-over-human-contact/
12. Cherry DK, Burt CW, Woodwell DA. National Ambulatory Medical Care Survey: 2001 summary: advance data from vital and health statistics. No. 337. Hyattsville MD: United States Department of Health and Human Services. 2003. Available at http://www.cdc.gov/nchs/data/ad/ad337.pdf
13. Bell DM, Gleiber DW, Mercer AA, et al. Illness associated with child day care: a study of incidence and cost. Am J Public Health. 1989;79:479–84.
14. Burke BL, Hall RW, Section on Telehealth Care. Telemedicine: pediatric applications. Pediatrics. 2015;136:e29. https://doi.org/10.1542/peds.2015-1517.
15. McConnochie KM. Potential of telemedicine in pediatric primary care. Pediatr Rev. 2006;27:e58. https://doi.org/10.1542/pir.27-9-e58.
16. The National Rural Health Association. Website. https://www.ruralhealthweb.org/about-nrha/about-rural-health-care. Accessed 30 Dec 2019.
17. National Advisory Committee on Rural Health and Human Services, Telehealth in Rural America. Policy Brief. March 2015. https://www.hrsa.gov/advisorycommittees/rural/publications/telehealthmarch2015.pdf
18. Dullet NW, Geraghty EM, Kaufman T, et al. Impact of a university-based outpatient telemedicine program on time savings, travel costs, and environmental pollutants. Value Health. 2017;20:542–6.

19. Hollander JE, Carr BG. Virtually perfect? Telemedicine for Covid-19. NEJM. 2020:1–3. https://doi.org/10.1056/NEJMp2003539.
20. Usher-Pines L, Fischer S, Ramya C. The promise of direct-to-consumer telehealth for disaster response and recovery. Prehospital and Disaster Med. 2016;31(4):454–6.
21. Murren-Boezem J, Solo-Josephson P, Zettler-Greeley CM. A pediatric telemedicine response to a natural disaster [published online ahead of print Sept 25 2019]. Telemed J E Health. 2019; https://doi.org/10.1089/tmj.2019.0100.
22. Lee KJ, Finnane A, Soyer HP. Recent trends in teledermatology and tele-dermoscopy. Dermatol Pract Concept. 2018;8(3):214–23.
23. Fogel AL, Sarin KY. A survey of direct-to-consumer teledermatology services available to US patients: explosive growth, opportunities and controversy. J Telemed Telecare. 2017;23(1):19–25.
24. Pande R, Morris M, Peters A, et al. Leveraging remote behavioral health interventions to improve medical outcomes and reduce costs. Am J Manag Care. 2015;21(2):e141–51.
25. Market Watch. Direct to consumer telehealth services – global market growth, opportunities, analysis of top key players and forecast to 2025. 2019. Accessible at https://www.marketwatch.com/press-release/global-direct-to-consumer-telehealth-services-market-2019-swot-analysis-seg-mentation-opportunities-and-forecast-to-2025-2019-02-28
26. J.D. Power. J.D. Power Telehealth Satisfaction Study; 2019. Accessible at https://www.jdpower.com/business/resource/us-telehealth-study
27. Halpren-Ruder D, Change AM, Hollander JE. Quality assurance in tele-health: adherence to evidence-based indicators. Telemed J E Health. 2018;25(7):599–604.
28. Pirtle C, Payne K, Telehealth DB. Legal and ethical considerations for success. Telehealth Med Today. 2019;4(144):1–6.
29. Brundisini F, Giacomini M, DeJean D, et al. Chronic disease patients' experiences with accessing health care in rural and remote areas: a systematic review and qualitative meta-synthesis. Ont Health Technol Assess Ser [Internet]. 2013; 13(15):1–33. Accessible at: http://www.hqontario.ca/en/documents/eds/2013/full-report-OCDM-rural-health-care.pdf
30. Bull TP, Dewar AR, Szalma JL. Considerations for the telehealth systems of tomorrow: an analysis of student perceptions of telehealth technologies. JMIR Med Educ. 2016;2(2):e11.
31. Uscher-Pines L, Mulcahy A, Cowling D, et al. Access and quality of care in direct-to-consumer telemedicine. Telemed J E Health. 2016;22(4):282–7.
32. Dinesen B, Nonnecke B, Lindeman D, et al. Personalized telehealth in the future: a global research agenda. J Med Internet Res. 2016;18(3):e53.
33. American Medical Association. Navigating state medical licensure. Website. Accessible at https://www.ama-assn.org/residents-students/career-planning-resource/navigating-state-medical-licensure

34. Interstate Medical Licensure Compact. Website. Accessible at https:// imlcc.org/
35. Elliott T, Shih J. Direct to consumer telemedicine. Curr Allergy Asthma Rep. 2019;19(1):1–5. Accessible at. https://doi.org/10.1007/s11882-019-0837-7.
36. Uscher-Pines L, Kahn J. Barriers and facilitators to pediatric emergency telemedicine in the United States. Telemed J E Health. 2014;20(11):990–6.
37. Ashwood JS, Mehrotra A, Cowling D, Uscher-Pines L. Direct to consumer telehealth may increase access to care but does not decrease spending. Health Aff. 2017;36(3):485–91.
38. Dorsey ER, Topol EJ. State of telehealth. N Engl J Med. 2016;375:154–61.
39. Zipnosis Survey. On-demand virtual care benchmark survey report; 2018. Accessible at https://www.zipnosis.com/wp-content/uploads/2019/03/2018-On-Demand-Virtual-Care-Benchmark-Survey-Report.pdf?utm_source=ATA+Website
40. Svorny SV. Liberating telemedicine: options to eliminate the state licensing roadblock. Cato Inst 2017;PA826. Accessible at https://www.cato.org/publications/policy-analysis/liberating-telemedicine-options-eliminate-state-licensing-roadblock
41. United States Department of Agriculture. USDA is investing in rural broadband. Website. Accessible at https://www.usda.gov/broadband

School-Based Telemedicine Services

12

Amanda Martin and Steve North

Caring for young orthopedic patients in the traditional outpatient setting may potentially result in a significant amount of missed school for students, missed work for parents, and a high rate of "no-show" visits for the practice. Providing orthopedic care for students while they're at school can benefit the patient, the family, and the practice in multiple ways. This chapter focuses on how to provide high-quality orthopedic and sports medicine care via the creation of a successful school-based telehealth program.

When considering the overall health of an adolescent, school attendance is essential for academic achievement and in turn high school graduation. High school graduation has a direct impact on long-term physical and emotional health of adolescents [1]. School-based health centers have been providing access to care at school for students for more than 35 years and have been shown to improve health outcomes and impact graduation rates [2]. There has been significant growth in the use of telehealth in schools over the past 10 years for acute, chronic, and follow-up care, and, with increased general acceptance of telehealth in

A. Martin (✉) · S. North
Center for Rural Health Innovation, Spruce Pine, NC, USA
e-mail: Amanda.martin@crhi.org; Steve.north@crhi.org

© Springer Nature Switzerland AG 2021
A. Atanda Jr., J. F. Lovejoy III (eds.), *Telemedicine in Orthopedic Surgery and Sports Medicine*,
https://doi.org/10.1007/978-3-030-53879-8_12

schools, there are many opportunities for orthopedic care [2]. Providing access to care at school, with needed imaging performed in advance at a convenient time for the student and family, can decrease absences and minimize the impact of an injury on academic achievement.

There are several different models that could be adopted or combined in the development of a school-based orthopedic and sports medicine telehealth program. Partnering with an existing school-based health center would allow for collaboration with a medical provider and nursing staff for the physical exam and arrangement of follow-up plans. Currently there are almost 11,000 school-based health centers in US public schools, and approximately 13% of US students have access to healthcare at school [2]. Collaborating with athletic trainers at a school allows a physician to expand how care is provided to students with acute injuries on the sidelines and with ongoing evaluation or rehabilitation from an injury. Another potential application is collaborating with physical therapists in the exceptional education program to treat students with congenital orthopedic issues [3].

Value to Students Students often miss post-injury follow-up visits due to multiple factors: a lack of transportation, a lack of understanding by the patient or the family regarding the importance of the appointment, and parents' inability to take additional time away from work, especially when they may have missed a significant amount of time to care for the initial injury. More frequent, shorter check-ins can increase adherence to a treatment plan, and by connecting with the patient at school, the school's involvement in the student's recovery can be improved.

Value to Providers Orthopedic and sports medicine practices often see a high rate of "no-show" visits among adolescent patients. Depending on the reasons, "no-shows" can be reduced dramatically by providing care in the school, where most students are legally required to be every weekday and public transportation is furnished. An additional potential benefit is the reputation of a practice is enhanced by making care easily accessible to patients.

Currently school-based telehealth is in the early stages of adoption, giving those providers who embrace it an edge in their community [4]. The financial and time investment to arrange a telehealth program is quickly returned with increased referrals, reduction of no-shows, and the marketing that is rolled into advertising the service. Additionally, by providing increased interaction with orthopedic surgeons and sports medicine physicians, athletic trainers at small or rural schools may have higher rates of confidence, job satisfaction, and retention.

School Value Proposition The value proposition to the school is essentially to reduce absenteeism for follow-up during a global recovery period. It is critical to build relationships in the schools that stress this most important point that care into the schools keeps the students there instead of in a waiting room at clinic. Public schools tend to be more receptive to programming that is equitable and available to all students, not only athletes. Injuries can happen in PE class, on the marching band field, and walking down the hallway. Additionally, there should be a plan for offering care to uninsured and underinsured patients as well. The schools should not have to accept financial liability for these students, but with an equity lens, underinsured and uninsured students should also have access. Sliding fee scales, hospital charity programs, and rational pre-set rates in addition to a plan for no-cost care will make a program proposal most appealing to a school.

What patients are suitable for telemedicine? Ultimately this is the decision of the individual practice, and the scope of practice may evolve over time as both the school and the orthopedic practice become more comfortable with using telehealth. Understanding the skill set of the presenter will have a direct impact on the types of visits seen. Several types of appointments are appropriate for school telehealth. Many patients do not require a hands-on evaluation by an orthopedic surgeon when they have a skilled presenter at the originating site. Simple injuries may be seen acutely or for follow-up with the school nurse as the presenter. Sports-related injuries, surgical follow-up visits, or an anomaly identified on a preparticipation physical, presented by an onsite athletic trainer, can easily be evaluated. Students with congenital diseases could be seen for evaluation of contractures or gait in combination with the physical therapist. If there is any concern whatsoever, there is always the option for the physician or advanced practitioner to ask the patient to come into the office to be seen in person.

As described in previous chapters, telehealth has requirements that make it different from providing care in person, in an outpatient clinic. Successful implementation of a school-based orthopedic and sports medicine telehealth program requires an application of a school lens onto the situation. The sections below outline key programmatic components that should be considered when approaching a school or school system. These should be combined with the previously mentioned value propositions in a comprehensive proposal. Each of these components should be considered prior to the first visit taking place. A clear memorandum of understanding outlining the expectations of both sides will increase the likelihood of a program's success.

Parental Consent Like all healthcare provided to minors, parental consent is a factor in school telehealth. It can sometimes be difficult, as a parent may not give consent in writing prior to an injury. Student athletes, especially if they are also receiving services from an athletic trainer or physical therapist on site, may already have a requirement for written consent from their parent/guardian, which could simply be modified to include physician care.

Information Sharing with the School The Family Education Rights and Privacy Act (FERPA) is the education system's privacy regulations rival HIPAA for complexity. FERPA outlines how a student's demographics, grades, attendance, discipline, and promotion records can be shared. An understanding of the balance between HIPAA and FERPA is essential because a telehealth presenter may be a school employee and therefore covered by FERPA. This limits what can be shared with whom on both sides of the telehealth encounter [5]. A clear data sharing agreement that addresses the needs of HIPAA and FERPA is a requirement of any school-based telehealth program.

Location   Location of the encounter within the school is another consideration. The space where the student is seen must be private from both visual and sound perspectives. To comply with HIPAA regulations, a visit with an injured high school athlete must be carried out in a private setting and not, for example, in a locker room. In addition to being a private space, the room may need to accommodate a wheelchair, a training table, and room to maneuver the telehealth equipment for a visit to be successful. The school nurse's office or the training room may be suitable locations.

Presenter   The presenter has multiple roles that include establishing the video connection, obtaining necessary vitals, introducing the patient, operating peripheral cameras as needed, assisting with the exam as appropriate based on training, scheduling follow-up, and coordinating communication with the school and family. In a school, the presenter may be a school nurse or aide, athletic trainer, coach, physical therapist, or a lay person. To some extent, this presenter is determined by the scope of services to be offered, for example, an athletic trainer is likely better able to assist in the initial evaluation of a possible knee ligament injury than the nurse's aide.

Technology   Engaging the school district's IT program early in the process of developing a school-based telehealth program will decrease frustrations with Internet connectivity during visits. Two key questions to ask are: (1) Can the school telehealth program connect to a school's existing Internet? (2) Are there technical specifications that need to be considered to allow the video signal to traverse the school's firewalls? This relationship is as important as the relationship developed with the school board and the principal.

Financials   Delivering orthopedic care via telehealth as a stand-alone program into a single school may be too cumbersome to be worthwhile. However, in combination with an onsite athletic trainer program or school-based health center, it can be an excellent opportunity for both the school and the orthopedic practice. Identify and develop these strategic entry points into the schools through the school nurse, school-based health center, or athletic trainer program.

References

1. Lee JO, Kosterman R, Jones TM, et al. Mechanisms linking high school graduation to health disparities in young adulthood: a longitudinal analysis of the role of health behaviours, psychosocial stressors, and health insurance. Public Health. 2016;139:61–9. https://doi.org/10.1016/j.puhe.2016.06.010.
2. Love HE, Schlitt J, Soleimanpour S, Panchal N, Behr C. Twenty years of school-based health care growth and expansion. Health Aff. 2019;38(5):755–64. https://doi.org/10.1377/hlthaff.2018.05472.
3. Gregory P, Alexander J, Satinsky J. Clinical telerehabilitation: applications for physiatrists. PM R. 2011;3(7):647–56. https://doi.org/10.1016/j.pmrj.2011.02.024.
4. Love H, Panchal N, Schlitt J, Behr C, Soleimanpour S. The use of telehealth in school-based health centers. Glob Pediatr Health. 2019;6:2333794X19884194. https://doi.org/10.1177/2333794X19884194.
5. Kiel JM, Knoblauch LM. HIPAA and FERPA: competing or collaborating? J Allied Health. 2010;39(4):e161–5.

Section III

Special Topics in Telemedicine

Telemedicine in a Time of Crisis: The COVID-19 Experience

13

John F. Lovejoy III and Patrick Barth

In March of 2020, it becomes apparent that cases of COVID-19 were rapidly increasing in the United States. Reports from other countries such as Italy elevated concerns that the United States was underestimating the potential impact of this pandemic. Many experts noted a lack of national, state, and institutional preparedness particularly with regard to critical care services, ICU capacity, and most importantly personal protective equipment. As a result, many hospital systems began decreasing access, limiting clinic services, and cancelling non-urgent/emergent surgeries. As families became increasingly concerned about entering healthcare facilities, the downstream effect resulted in delays in non-urgent and urgent care for patients, the underevaluation and treatment of identified problems, and severe financial stress for hospital

J. F. Lovejoy III (✉)
Department of Orthopaedics, Sports Medicine and Physical Medicine and Rehabilitation, University of Central Florida School of Medicine, Nemours Children's Hospital, Orlando, FL, USA
e-mail: John.Lovejoy@nemours.org

P. Barth
Division of Otolaryngology, Department of Surgery, Nemours/Alfred I. duPont Hospital for Children, Wilmington, DE, USA
e-mail: pbarth@nemours.org

© Springer Nature Switzerland AG 2021
A. Atanda Jr., J. F. Lovejoy III (eds.), *Telemedicine in Orthopedic Surgery and Sports Medicine*,
https://doi.org/10.1007/978-3-030-53879-8_13

139

systems. Clinical and administrative leadership were thrust into an unprecedented situation.

One proposed solution for clinical care was the utilization of telemedicine. Prior to COVID-19, use of telemedicine in orthopedics was limited. On an institutional level, a telehealth structure was in place but had only been utilized across the enterprise in a limited fashion. Senior leadership started to make preparations for widespread clinical disruption. A task force was assigned with leaders from across the organization with the telehealth team integrated into this group to help support the health system. The primary goal was to help support primary care, and urgent care, because it was felt this would feel the initial surge of ill patients and could quickly be overwhelmed. As an organization, this was already established, as there was a well-established 24/7 on-demand urgent care platform.

In a parallel fashion, there was a similar focus on specialty care. Specialty care had the advantage as many providers had already adopted telemedicine at least in part into their practice. Each specialty division was reviewed to make sure at least one provider was previously trained and enrolled in the online platform. For larger divisions, more than one provider was identified. Orthopedics were early adopters with several champions who already had demonstrated successful use cases. A recent experiment with a dedicated clinic had identified barriers with provider training, patient scheduling systems, and the reliability of the technology primarily on the patient side. These findings were not only true on the department level, but throughout the enterprise.

As cases started to rise in the United States and specifically in Florida and New York, the need for restricted travel and social distancing were becoming increasingly apparent. Although our institution is solely pediatric, concerns were raised that we needed to prepare for a possible surge and potentially may be required to accommodate adult patients if adult institutions reached capacity. As in-person clinics began to shut down and in order to further minimize direct contact, an essential component of social distancing, the department reengaged the idea of telemedicine. The first step was to identify a telemedicine champion to lead the team and then initiate training for all providers, as all providers now wanted access to the platform. This was a very large task as it took approximately 20 minutes to enroll each provider on the platform, and then all these providers needed training. This was true for over 600 providers across the hospital system.

The orthopedic department leveraged their prior experience, and a dedicated telemedicine clinic was then established each day Monday–Friday. Initially most telemedicine patients were less complicated non-urgent problems, such as range of motion checks, simple wound checks, and reviewing results from previously ordered advanced imaging studies.

As the concern over the pandemic intensified, we began expanding the limits of our telemedicine use to areas traditionally reserved for in-person visits. The department began to triage urgent but non-emergent patients, such as those with less complicated fractures, to confirm whether or not an in-person visit was warranted. When the determination was made that an in-person visit was required, the information gathered during the triage process allowed for better preparation for the follow-up appointment. In some situations, patients or their families only need to stop by the clinic to obtain a piece of DME. In other cases, where a more involved work-up required additional services such as radiographs, fracture reduction, or casting, the visits were organized in advance to maximize the safety of the patient, the provider, and the clinic staff. By mid-April, the Department of Orthopedics had completely embraced telemedicine. The lessons learned through this experience can be applied to future crisis, particularly those that limit direct in-person consumer access to healthcare resources.

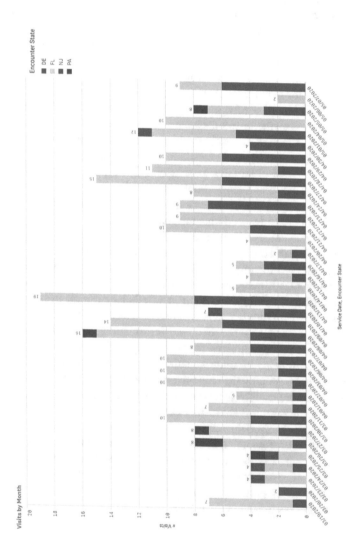

Key Points when Using Telemedicine in a Crisis Situation

- Initial setup
    - Designate a champion for telemedicine who will become your team's expert.
    - Use the designated champion to facilitate training for all providers as quickly as possible.
    - Pick a platform that provides appropriate HIPAA compliance from phones and tablets as providers will need the flexibility of a mobile platform to perform visits from non-traditional settings (i.e., home). Have a backup plan if technical challenges prohibit the primary modality.
    - Evaluate and/or designate each provider's mode of providing visits.
        Type of device the provider will utilize: computer, tablet, or phone
        Location of the provider when they perform the visits and the quality of bandwidth
    - Use a video-capable system.
        Video brings in a greater level of personnel contact and can build a stronger physician-patient relationship.
        Can be utilized to allow the provider to visually assess the patient's home environment. This may change the treatment plan (i.e., house with many tight corridors may not allow a wheelchair, a high number of steps may impede mobility, etc.).
        Interaction with a medical provider by video allows both the medical provider and the family to use the power of body and facial gestures to provide a more in-depth connection. This is particularly powerful in a crisis situation where providers can assess for secondary issues that may be impacting their patients such as isolation and unhealthy levels of stress.
    - Consider needs of families, such as access to technology, Internet access, and availability of interpreter services.
    - Visits need detailed instructions or support staff contacting the families to assist in preparation for their visit.

- Conducting the visit
  - During the scheduling process, clearly set expectations for patient/family behavior during the visit.

    Patient/family should be appropriately dressed for the visit.

    For minors, family should stay present and engaged for the entire visit.
  - Reiterate behavioral expectations, if violated, and if necessary, terminate the visit.
  - Have a medical assistant (MA, nurse, PA) available to be present for the visit if it may entail the examination of any compromising part of the body (wound check around genitalia or the buttocks, etc.)
  - Remind patients/families not to conduct a visit while driving a vehicle or while performing other tasks for which their attention must have precedence.
- Using telemedicine for triage
  - In a crisis situation, telemedicine can be an excellent option to triage patients and determine the need for possible transfer from outside institutions.
  - Pearls for using telemedicine for triage

    Expectations are important. Set the expectation at the time of scheduling that the patient may need to have a second in-person visit. Remind the patient/family of this possibility at the beginning of the actual visit.

    Have a definitive plan in place for those patients that are determined to need an in-person visit.

    Depending on insurance, patients/families may incur two copays for the "initial" evaluation of the problem.

    Many new patient visits require radiographs for assessment. If feasible, arrange for the patient to obtain them prior to the visit. Those who are unable to obtain radiographs prior to the visit should be seen in person at a location that can perform the radiographs.
- Other uses
  - During a crisis, patients/family may be limited in their ability, or due to travel restrictions, from participating in thera-

peutic services ordered by your service. Telemedicine visits can be used to give patient home therapy instructions and to monitor their therapy progress.

- Selling points to patients/families
  - No need for transportation (many of our patients are dependent on Medicaid transport which may be affected in a crisis)
  - Easy and quick to answer questions regarding unexpected problems without leaving home (i.e., post-op dressing and wound issues)
  - Minimizes the impact on parent/family work schedule
  - Decreased exposure for family, provider, and support staff
- Challenges/barriers
  - Connectivity issues as Internet reliability and strength are variable for many patients.
  - Families misunderstanding the log-in process resulting in visit delays and sometimes requiring the original visit to be cancelled and a new visit to be entered into the system.
  - Families prematurely ending visits.
  - Difficulty with lab and therapy orders. In our system, these orders could not be placed by telemedicine, and an RN in one of our offices had to place the orders.
  - Limited ability to perform physical exams and to review radiographs.
  - No ability to perform radiographs.
- Other pearls
  - Streamline and simplify your scheduling process. Questions to ask:
    - Are there certain visit types for which you can mandate telemedicine?
    - Are there certain visit types for which telemedicine will not work?
  - Our staff has anecdotally noticed that families seem to be more engaged in the telemedicine follow-up visits compared with equivalent in-person visits. Reasons heard by families for this improved engagement included less stress over needing to "be somewhere after the visit," follow-up visits

are less stressful in general than the uncertainty embedded in a new patient visit, and the security of performing the visit in the "safe" environment of their home increased their comfort level.

- Post-op wound checks can be excellent telemedicine visits; however, certain wounds are more challenging such as complex foot, hip, and spine wounds.
- Remember to use a staff member chaperone for the visit when appropriate.
- Create a telehealth inbox (email address) to provide a centralized platform for patients to send follow-up questions.

Global Telemedicine Health and Educational Initiatives

14

Rameez Qudsi, Carlos Pargas,
and Emmanuel Opati

Overview

The very nature of telehealth, utilizing technology to bridge gaps in distance and time, makes it uniquely amenable to international use. Recognizing the potential value of such applications, the World Health Organization (WHO), as part of the larger United Nations (UN) Sustainable Development Goals, has made eHealth a core component of its efforts toward universal health coverage. It has been implementing a focused strategy since 2005, including the development of a Global Observatory to study and disseminate knowledge on eHealth throughout the 194 member nations.

In 2016, the WHO concluded its report on the Third Global Survey of eHealth documenting areas of progress as well as ongoing need in the dissemination of global technology aimed toward improving health. They reiterate the broad definition of eHealth as

R. Qudsi (✉) · C. Pargas
Department of Orthopaedics, Nemours/A.I. duPont Hospital for
Children, Wilmington, DE, USA
e-mail: qudsi@post.harvard.edu; Carlos.Pargas@nemours.org

E. Opati
XpertCare Inc., Baltimore, MD, USA
e-mail: emmanuelopati@xpertcare.online

© Springer Nature Switzerland AG 2021   147
A. Atanda Jr., J. F. Lovejoy III (eds.), *Telemedicine in Orthopedic Surgery and Sports Medicine*,
https://doi.org/10.1007/978-3-030-53879-8_14

"the cost-effective and secure use of information communication technologies (ICT) in support of health and health-related fields, including health-care services, health surveillance, health literature, and health education, knowledge and research." Telehealth, an evolving core component of eHealth, is now promoted by the WHO as "the delivery of health care services, where patients and providers are separated by distance. Telehealth uses ICT for the exchange of information for the diagnosis and treatment of diseases and injuries, research and evaluation, and for the continuing education of health professionals. Telehealth can contribute to achieving universal health coverage by improving access for patients to quality, cost-effective, health services wherever they may be. It is particularly valuable for those in remote areas, vulnerable groups and ageing populations" [1]. Importantly, these definitions highlight both clinical services for patients and ongoing education for healthcare providers.

Clinical Applications

Perhaps the most apparent clinical application of telehealth in an international context is to improve access to care for patients both within and across national borders. Types of clinical care can be distinguished based on utilization in high-income developed nations versus that in low- to middle-income developing nations. In both settings, telemedicine can be applied to extend the reach of clinicians from urban centers to rural, less populated parts of a country.

In high-income countries, telemedicine often manifests as specialists in cities and/or academic centers providing consultation services to frontline healthcare workers in rural areas. A governmental telehealth system is utilized in Canada, for example, to reach patients in the remote Yukon region. Mobile telehealth units in community health centers are used to access physicians in the cities, with patients and providers agreeing that these services improve timely access and reduce cost but remain underutilized [2]. A broad array of telehealth applications to service remote and rural areas is also seen in Australia, where over 70 such programs have been identified, increasing exponentially since 2010 [3]. In addition to physician services, telehealth has been demonstrated to provide value in extending the services of allied health professionals (e.g., therapists, nurses, psychologists, social workers, dieticians, pharmacists) to remote areas [4].

In low- to middle-income countries (LMIC), however, with many fewer physicians per capita and particularly low diffusion of providers to rural areas, telemedicine is used to improve access not just to specialists but also general doctors, nurses, and allied health professionals. Such projects have taken many different forms, at varying levels of sophistication, in developing nations [5]. One example of a large, well-developed program is the expansive telemedicine network established in India through the Apollo Hospital Group and other national institutions, to connect villages with district hospitals and urban specialty centers. The program has even explored collaboration with the Indian Space Research Organization for a dedicated healthcare satellite to support such efforts [6]. These telehealth networks in low-resource nations can involve direct provider-to-patient interaction as well as provider-to-provider consultation and education (see Chap. 11 on Provider-to-Provider telehealth applications).

In addition to "within-country" services, telemedicine strategies offer clinicians in low-resource countries the opportunity to engage with providers and healthcare systems in other higher-income nations to increase and improve clinical care in resource-poor settings. This can complement in-person visits by foreign teams and be a means for clinical case review and consultation and/or a mechanism for continuing medical education. Traditional "mission trip" style global health programs can be expanded using telehealth approaches to include clinical follow-up and outcome research after visiting healthcare providers return to their home country. This can allay some of the clinical and ethical concerns of short-term, infrequent trips to developing countries by providing important follow-up as well as maintaining relationships with local providers. Some groups even continue teaching and building local capacity with telehealth-assisted surgeries in the form of live assistance and feedback during a broadcasted surgical procedure by a local physician. This supports local physician education, broadens access to care, and provides opportunity for education for others observing the broadcast procedure.

Physicians in developed nations can also engage in ongoing case reviews with their colleagues in low-resource nations, using a variety of Internet-based platforms to share patient histories, physical exam findings, and relevant imaging. Such activities serve both direct clinical and educational purposes. This type of case review and consultation can be synchronous when technology and physician schedules allow but more feasibly may be conducted in an asynchronous manner. The Boston Children's Hospital Vascular Anomalies Center, for example, has a long-standing weekly multidisciplinary conference to review cases from around the world, submitted and reviewed in an asynchronous manner. Global physicians contact the Center and submit cases through an online portal, and once all appropriate notes and studies are collected by program staff, the consulting group meets to provide feedback on differential diagnoses and treatment options and, based on resources available near the patient, may either guide local care or provide a recommendation to travel to the United States [7]. This format not only provides critical advising with minimal delays but also acts as a method of screening to prevent unnecessary travel for patients and families.

Educational Applications

As part of the WHO definition, a key component of telehealth is the use of ICT for ongoing education of health professionals. With advances in communications technology platforms, and an increasingly high rate of access to telecommunications devices around the world, even in low-resource settings, teaching in medicine can go beyond traditional models of local, in-person, real-time encounters. Videoconferencing, online lectures, live surgery broadcasts, and virtual case discussions are just a few of the many potential global applications of telehealth in education.

Education among healthcare professionals is perhaps the most immediately accessible and common type of telehealth education. Medical lectures and skills demonstrations are essential to training others but can be extended to an international audience using both synchronous and asynchronous technologies. One example of such an initiative developed by the Geneva University Hospitals is through their RAFT (Réseau en Afrique Francophone pour la Télémédecine) network of eHealth across at least ten French-speaking nations in Africa [8]. The program incorporates interactive courses webcast across the network, as well as discussion of clinical cases across different countries [9].

Telehealth education can also be leveraged within a country, embedded within networks of telemedicine aimed at assisting healthcare providers in rural areas with subspecialty support. Project ECHO (Extension for Community Healthcare Outcomes) is a well-developed example begun in the United States in 2003 to extend hepatitis C expertise to rural areas in the state of New Mexico [10]. It was designed as a hub-and-spokes model of education for regular interactive videoconference didactic teaching sessions and reviews of de-identified patient cases, connecting specialists in the university setting with rural clinicians. Since then, the model has evolved to a more weblike network of specialists, extended to other clinical problems like osteoporosis management, and expanded to other countries like Ireland and Russia. Importantly, the group demonstrated benefits of academic study of the effort, showing a reduction in adverse events among a prospective group of patients with hepatitis C at Project ECHO sites compared to patients at sites not connected with the network. Such work enabled the proposal of formal legislation through the US Congress to study and fund telehealth education and can be a model for public-private partnerships in expanding access to medical education using technology.

An illustrative example of a pediatric-specific program modeled after ECHO is Specialist Access to Children Everywhere (SpACE) at Texas Children's Hospital in the United States. This program brings together general pediatricians from the community and pediatric subspecialists for a weekly patient case review. The goal of the program is to make subspecialists more available in a structured format to answer questions from referring pediatricians. It is designed so that as a subspecialist answers a clinical question, other pediatricians in the network also learn from it, with both pros and cons to this format (Table 14.1). With such a group education model, over time one hope is to reduce the volume and delay of back-and-forth phone calls between subspecialists and referring pediatricians. Although still in its pilot phase, the program provides some lessons that can be shared with other clinicians considering a similar model.

In addition to continuing education for healthcare providers, eHealth technologies can be used for direct-to-patient, or population, healthcare education. Given the broad reach of mobile phones and telecommunication even in developing countries,

Table 14.1 Pros and cons of the SpACE model of clinical and educational telehealth conferencing between pediatricians and subspecialists. This model can be applied globally between primary care providers and specialists and also between healthcare educators and trainees

Pros	Cons
Structured format: The schedule and case for discussion can be agreed upon ahead of time, for example, case discussion every Wednesday at 8:00 am–8:15 am. Case for the week sent out to the group prior to the day of the event. This allows for structure and time commitment needed by clinicians.	Pediatricians are likely to attend sessions when they have a specific question about their patients for the specialists. They are less likely to attend and benefit from a discussion on another clinician's patient, especially if there are time conflicts with other commitments.
Flexibility: Invited clinicians can attend the session from anywhere if they have access to any mobile device with Internet connection. Also, when sessions are recorded, clinicians unable to attend the real-time case discussion can view it later.	Pediatricians are unlikely to watch the case discussion later if it is not about their patient. Availability of the recorded video makes it another webinar, of which there are many of those.
Access point to subspecialists: Given that face-to-face interactions between pediatricians and subspecialists are infrequent, virtual case discussions present an opportunity for clinicians to put a face to the names and thereby strengthen professional relationships.	Subspecialists may be put on the spot semi-publicly with questions they are unprepared for. However, as professional relationships build, this becomes less of a concern, and questions can be deferred from one session to the next to allow an adequate and researched response.

many groups have attempted to leverage these tools in increasing public awareness and knowledge surrounding health. A review of text messaging-based programs identified over 30 different programs in low-resource settings using SMS for population-level medical advocacy, education, and care [11]. Multiple programs were focused on HIV/AIDS and sexual and reproductive awareness and education. In addition, programs were implemented for SMS-based healthcare tips and information surrounding general health as well as specific diseases in times of crisis such as the cholera outbreak in Zimbabwe and the SARS epidemic in China. Such low-tech, population-level innovations can offer critical information and advocacy to those otherwise not able to access healthcare providers.

Summary and Implications

The very nature of telemedicine reduces the impact of distance and geography on access to healthcare services. Global health, therefore, becomes a natural area of medicine amenable to telehealth applications. This highlights the need for ongoing development in legal and professional standards for physicians and healthcare staff to engage more readily across traditional boundaries of state or country. Furthermore, there must be increased effort by governments and private global communities to bolster technological infrastructure in low-resource settings to ensure access to this growing mode of healthcare. In 2018, WHO member states at the 71st World Health Assembly unanimously endorsed a resolution recognizing the importance of government support for digital health toward achieving universal healthcare coverage, a core component of the UN Sustainable Development Goals [12]. Analysis of the prior WHO Global Survey on eHealth demonstrates that a country's commitment to digital health innovation is a stronger metric of national progress than absolute income or healthcare expenditure, giving hope for the future of ICT and telemedicine in all nations despite great differences in GDP [13]. Perhaps digital health can in fact help level the playing field in a world of otherwise increasing economic inequalities.

Beyond the immediate benefits of clinical care, continuing medical education, and cost savings, the use of telehealth in global health fields can also have broader implications on volunteerism. A survey of volunteers at a telemedicine clinic in the United States offering services to LMIC demonstrated time constraints as a major barrier to volunteerism but increased direct patient interaction and engagement as primary motivator [14]. Telemedicine platforms are uniquely suited to allow volunteer physicians to reach patients and healthcare professionals in LMIC without the relatively high time commitment of international travel, thus encouraging greater volunteerism. In addition, for those providers who do continue to travel, telemedicine services can be used to continue clinical care and follow-up of their own patients in their country of origin. In this way, global physician volunteer work can be less disruptive financially and logistically to one's normal clinical practice and ongoing patient care needs.

As telecommunications technology advances at a rapid rate, opportunities for telemedicine applications in global health will only increase with time. Two-way communication and long-term partnerships can be developed in these ways to improve access to medical care and education even to the most remote parts of the globe. By continuing to innovate and study international digital health applications, the field of global health can move beyond intermittent, limited encounters to more sustainable, high-impact methods of expanding access to care around the world.

References

1. World Health Organization. Global diffusion of eHealth: making universal health coverage achievable, Report of the third global survey on eHealth. December 2016. ISBN: 978-92-4-151178-0. Available publicly at: https://www.who.int/goe/publications/global_diffusion/en/
2. Seto E, Smith D, Jacques M, Morita PP. Opportunities and challenges of telehealth in remote communities: case study of the Yukon telehealth system. JMIR Med Inform. 2019;7(4):e11353.
3. Bradford NK, Caffery LJ, Smith AC. Telehealth services in rural and remote Australia: a systematic review of models of care and factors influencing success and sustainability. Rural Remote Health. 2016;16(4):4268.

4. Speyer R, Denman D, Wilkes-Gillan S, Chen YW, Bogaardt H, Kim JH, Heckathorn DE, Cordier R. Effects of telehealth by allied health professionals and nurses in rural and remote areas: a systematic review and meta-analysis. J Rehabil Med. 2018;50(3):225–35.
5. Combi C, Pozzani G, Pozzi G. Telemedicine for developing countries. A survey and some design issues. Appl Clin Inform. 2016;7(4):1025–50.
6. Bagchi S. Telemedicine in rural India. PLoS Med. 2006;3(3):e82.
7. Boston Children's Hospital, Vascular Anomalies Center, VAC Conference. http://www.childrenshospital.org/centers-and-services/programs/o-_-z/vascular-anomalies-center-program/programs-and-services/vac-conference. Accessed Jan 2020.
8. Bagayoko CO, Müller H, Geissbuhler A. Assessment of internet-based tele-medicine in Africa (the RAFT project). Comput Med Imaging Graph. 2006;30(6–7):407–16.
9. Geissbuhler A, Bagayoko CO, Ly O. The RAFT network: 5 years of distance continuing medical education and tele-consultations over the Internet in French-speaking Africa. Int J Med Inform. 2007;76(5–6):351–6.
10. Lewiecki EM, Jackson A 3rd, Lake AF, Carey JJ, Belaya Z, Melnichenko GA, Rochelle R. Bone health TeleECHO: a force multiplier to improve the care of skeletal diseases in underserved communities. Curr Osteoporos Rep. 2019;17(6):474–82.
11. Déglise C, Suggs LS, Odermatt P. Short message service (SMS) applications for disease prevention in developing countries. J Med Internet Res. 2012;14(1):e3.
12. Labrique A, Vasudevan L, Mehl G, Rosskam E, Hyder AA. Digital health and health systems of the future. Glob Health Sci Pract. 2018;6(Suppl 1):S1–4.
13. Novillo-Ortiz D, Dumit EM, D'Agostino M, et al. Digital health in the Americas: advances and challenges in connected health. BMJ Innov. 2018;4(3):123–7.
14. Kim EJ, Fox S, Moretti ME, Turner M, Girard TD, Chan SY. Motivations and barriers associated with physician volunteerism for an international telemedicine organization. Front Public Health. 2019;7:224.

Telemedicine Research and Quality Assessment

15

Judd E. Hollander and Jason Goldwater

Over the past decade, there has been a shift toward redesigning healthcare delivery to be more patient-centered, convenient, and cost-effective [1–4]. Telehealth, or telemedicine, is increasingly used as a means of providing patient-centered care. Telehealth includes telecommunication via a variety of different platforms, facilitating care that can be delivered to patients when and where they choose to receive it [5–7]. The Health Resources and Services Administration (HRSA) has defined it as "the use of electronic information and telecommunications technologies to support and promote long-distance clinical healthcare, patient and professional health-related education, public health and health administration" [8].

J. E. Hollander (✉)
Healthcare Delivery Innovation, Thomas Jefferson University, Philadelphia, PA, USA

Strategic Health Initiatives, Sidney Kimmel Medical College, Philadelphia, PA, USA

Finance and Healthcare Enterprises, Department of Emergency Medicine, Sidney Kimmel Medical College, Philadelphia, PA, USA

J. Goldwater
Atlas Research, LLC, Washington, DC, USA

© Springer Nature Switzerland AG 2021
A. Atanda Jr., J. F. Lovejoy III (eds.), *Telemedicine in Orthopedic Surgery and Sports Medicine*,
https://doi.org/10.1007/978-3-030-53879-8_15

Telehealth has been used in a variety of surgical settings as a means of connecting patients, providers, and family members. Examples of clinical uses include many forms of synchronous and asynchronous care such as the provision of remote specialist consults, provider-to-provider training, bringing services to rural communities, direct patient-provider communication through asynchronous platforms (text messaging or e-mail communications) or direct face-to-face video connections, and monitoring of patients at home. Telemedicine has been used in the preoperative, operative, and postoperative setting.

Telemedicine is just a means to an end. Telemedicine is not really about the technology; it is better thought of as a different form of healthcare delivery. The care needed and care delivered need to be tailored to the patients' medical or surgical condition and needs. It improves access by bringing care to the patients when and where they need it. Orthopedic surgeons may provide remote services in a variety of settings such as emergency departments, urgent care or occupational medicine clinics, hospital wards, homes, and at disaster sites [9–18].

As telemedicine is relatively new, there are overarching concerns regarding the quality of telehealth services and whether it provides the same level of care to that of in-person care. Of course, that might depend upon the particular patient, the patient's condition, location, and access to timely orthopedic assessment and definitive care. Fundamentally, we believe that telemedicine research should focus on the items important to the care of the patient with the specific condition. Thus, whether the patient is treated in person or via telemedicine, the assessment should be the same. Additionally, as telemedicine is just one form of a care delivery model in someone receiving or providing longitudinal care, research projects may be better suited to evaluate care of the patient with "x" via standard mechanism versus care of the patient with "x" with both standard of care and telemedicine.

When beginning a telemedicine program, internally, as with every clinical program, it is important to have established quality metrics and track success for telemedicine programs. New programs often focus on measures of adoption which may include:

- Number of app downloads

- Number of patient registrations
- Patient experience (satisfaction) reports or scores
- Number or proportion of providers trained
- Provider utilization
- Provider experience/satisfaction, as assessed by formal surveys
- Platform performance (audio-video connectivity rates)
- Number of telemedicine encounters
- Number of repeat visits
- New customer acquisition

More mature programs will align their metrics to national quality standards. It is national quality standards that inform pay for performance metrics, develop bundles, and lead to changes in outcomes for our patients. We recommend aligning research questions with the outcomes incorporated into national quality standards, recognizing this is only one potential approach.

The National Quality Forum (NQF) [19] recently developed a measure framework to create metrics to assess the use and effectiveness of telehealth services across multiple clinical settings, including out-of-hospital, ambulatory, emergency department, and within-hospital settings in rural, suburban, and urban areas. The framework was designed to serve as a foundation that identifies measures and measure concepts and services to assess the quality of care provided using telehealth modalities.

NQF began the project by conducting a comprehensive environmental scan to identify existing measures related to the use of telehealth in multiple clinical settings. Information was gathered through a multitude of sources, including documents published by operating divisions within HHS and other federal departments, such as the Department of Veterans Affairs (VA) and Department of Defense (DoD). These also include vendor-based white papers and reports issued by nonprofit organizations such as the American Telemedicine Association (ATA), the National Association for Community Health Centers (NACHC), the National Association of Rural Health Providers (NARHP), and the Health Information Management and Systems Society (HIMSS). Papers reviewed from various divisions of HHS – such as the Assistant Secretary for Planning and Evaluation (ASPE), Agency for Healthcare Research and Quality (AHRQ), and the Office of the National Coordinator for Health Information Technology (ONC) – included several published telehealth documents, such as ASPE's 2016 Report to Congress: E-health and Telemedicine and the 2016 Federal Telehealth Compendium.

The results of the environmental scan helped organize ideas and provide high-level guidance and direction on telehealth measurement priorities and their impact on healthcare delivery and outcomes. The central organizing principle of the framework was that the use of various telehealth modalities provides healthcare services to those who may not otherwise receive them in a timely effective manner. The use of telehealth does not represent a different type of healthcare within clinical settings, such as emergency departments, but rather a different method of healthcare delivery that provides services that are either similar in both scope and outcome or supplemental to those provided during an in-person encounter. The domains identified by NQF environmental scan are directly relevant to quality and research needs within orthopedics (Table 15.1).

As telemedicine programs expand, research and quality metrics should be tied to specific use cases and may include items like:

- Time from first contact to visit completion with decreased travel requirements
- New customer acquisition that might result from expanding geographic reach for preoperative assessment and postoperative care
- Readmission avoidance through the use of telemedicine
- Decreased cost of care in bundles that included telemedicine versus those that do not

The NQF final report, *Creating a Framework to Support Measure Development for Telehealth* [7], provides a framework

Table 15.1 Classification areas of information for the National Quality Forum environmental scan [19]

Domains	Potential information
Access to care	Timely receipt of health services Access to health services for those living in rural and urban communities Access to health services for those living in medically underserved areas Access to appropriate health specialists based on the need of the patient Increased provider capacity Access to patients that need specialized healthcare services
Cost	The costs of telehealth for public and private payers Efficient use of services for the patient Difference in cost per service and/or episode of care
Cost-effectiveness	Effect of telehealth on patient self-management Reduction in medical errors Reduction in overuse of services Cost savings to patient, family, and caregivers related to travel and time away from work
Patient experience	Appropriateness of services Increase in patient's knowledge of care Patient compliance with care regimens Difference in morbidity/mortality among specific clinical areas Shared decision-making Whether the care provided is safe, effective, patient-centered, timely, efficient, and equitable
Clinician experience	Diagnostic accuracy of telehealth applications Ability to obtain actionable information (enough to inform decision-making) Comfort with telehealth applications and procedures Quality of communications with patients Satisfaction with delivery method Impact on practice patterns

for telehealth measurement organized into four main domains (Table 15.2). Quality of care crosses all of these domains (e.g., untimely care represents poor-quality care, and ineffective care represents low-quality care).

Table 15.2 Domains and subdomains of the National Quality Forum telehealth measurement framework [19]

Domain	Subdomain(s)
Access to care	Access for patient, family, and/or caregiver Access for care team Access to information
Financial impact/cost	Financial impact to patient, family, and/or caregiver Financial impact to care team Financial impact to health system or payer Financial impact to society
Experience	Patient, family, and/or caregiver experience Care team member experience Community experience
Effectiveness	System effectiveness Clinical effectiveness Operational effectiveness Technical effectiveness

Access to care specifically is meant to address whether the use of telehealth services allows remote individuals to obtain clinical services effectively. With respect to orthopedics, it is essential to evaluate access across five major areas:

1. Affordability – Are both patients and members of the care team willing to accept the potential costs of telehealth as opposed to the alternative of not receiving or delivering traditional orthopedic care at all or receiving delayed care? What is the cost of providing telehealth services to those in need of care, and what is its effect on hospitals and ambulatory practices?

2. Availability – Does a telehealth modality provide access to a specialist that can provide care required by the patient, when it is requested or desired by the patient?

3. Accessibility – Is the technology necessary for an urgent, emergent, or elective telehealth consultation accessed and used by members of the care team?

4. Accommodation – Do the various modalities of telehealth accommodate the diverse needs of patients seeking emergency

care? Are patients able to access personnel through telehealth when requested?

5. Acceptability – Do both patients and care providers accept the use of telehealth as a means of care delivery?

Access to care includes not just access for patient but also access for family, and/or caregiver [20], and access for physicians and other care providers. Access for the patient, family, and/or caregiver refers to the ability of patients to receive services from providers they could not access otherwise because of geographical barriers and other logistical difficulties (such as transportation and travel costs) [21, 22]. Access for providers and other clinical staff means they have appropriate access to telehealth technologies to provide treatment when needed. For example, the access to a modality such as video teleconferencing provides a method for providers and emergency medical technicians to provide specific guidance to patients with emergency conditions.

Financial impact/cost of telehealth services includes financial impact to patient, family, and/or caregiver; financial impact to care team; financial impact to health system or payer; and financial impact to society. The financial impact to a patient, family, and/or caregiver accounts for the potential cost savings and benefits of telehealth such as less travel time to see a provider and more appropriate levels of care for a patient seeking orthopedic services. The financial impact to care providers and the patient includes the opportunity costs and both direct and indirect costs associated with providing care using a telehealth modality. The financial impact to payers and health systems includes cost avoidance and opportunity costs. The financial impact to society includes the impact of telehealth on healthcare workforce shortages, impact on hospitals of services provided at a distance, overall health status of a community, economic productivity, patient-provider convenience, and averted care.

Experience represents the usability and effect of telehealth on patients, care team members, and community at large and whether the use of telehealth resulted in a level of care that individuals and providers expected. For patients, family, and/or caregivers, experience refers to their ability to use the technology, the provision of a mechanism to connect with an emergency provider when needed, and whether the care delivered through various telehealth modalities is comparable to the quality of the care services they would receive during an in-person encounter [23, 24].

Patient and provider experience (rather than just satisfaction) are important quality components and require special attention in telemedicine since direct in-person patient-provider contact is lacking. Satisfaction with the technological aspects of the interaction should be separated from that of the provider. Since interacting with a patient over telemedicine requires some differences in interaction, such as eye contact, environment, and audio-video quality, these aspects should be monitored. How to best train providers in web-side manner and telemedicine-based evaluations is an area ripe for research [25, 26].

Effectiveness should include system, clinical, operational, and technical aspects of telehealth. System effectiveness refers to the ability of a telehealth modality and the overall system to assist in the coordination of care across various healthcare settings; to assist providers in discerning between urgent and non-urgent care; and to facilitate the sharing of information between providers to aid in decision-making. Clinical effectiveness refers to the impact of telehealth on health outcomes well as the comparative effectiveness of services provided in person. Operational effectiveness revolves around how clinically integrated telehealth is within the care setting. Technical effectiveness refers to the ability of the telehealth system to record and transmit images, data, and other information accurately to members of the care team, as well as the system's ability to exchange information between stakeholders seamlessly. All of these areas are ripe for research.

Outcome measures should depend upon the specific application of telemedicine. Some examples are mortality, frequency of prescriptions such as antibiotics, testing ordered, or frequency of clinical worsening requiring an in-person visit or hospitalization.

Research Tips

Clinical trial and research design are beyond the scope of this chapter. You can't learn them in a book. We recommend that those of you who plan to do research to evaluate telehealth focus on the domains specified by NQF [27].

Remember that telemedicine is just one type of care delivery, received by some patients, some of the time. Therefore, comparison of care pathways with and without telemedicine might be more important than comparing single encounters with telemedicine to single in-person encounters. Also, please make sure that comparisons of care including telemedicine are with the patient's best options, which sometimes might be no care. Only comparing telemedicine to in-person care ignores the 20–30% of patients who might not have access or need to cancel their appointment for logistical concerns. The NQF measures are likely to be universally adopted, and therefore mature programs should be encouraged to measure and report quality outcomes in alignment with these recommendations. The four domains in the NQF report have already been incorporated into research in primary care and internal medicine [23, 24], urology [28], general surgery [29], otolaryngology [30], preadmission testing [18], and oncology [27].

We recommend incorporation into the practice of and study of orthopedics. In this manner, we are able to determine the use and effectiveness of telehealth as a means of standard orthopedic care.

References

1. Committee on Quality of Health Care in America – Institute of Medicine. Crossing the quality chasm a new health system for the 21st century. Washington, DC: National Academy Press; 2001. http://www.iom.edu/ Reports/2001/Crossing-the-Quality-Chasm-A-New-Health-System-for-the-21st-Century.aspx. Accessed 9 Jan 2014.
2. Hickam D, Totten A, Berg A, Rader K, Goodman S, Newhouse R. The PCORI methodology report PCORI Methodology Committee. 2013 November.
3. Hollander JE, Davis TM, Doarn C, Goldwater JC, Klasko S, Lowery C, Papanagnou D, Rasmussen P, Sites FD, Stone D, Carr BG. Recommendations from the first National Academic Consortium of telehealth. Popul Health Manag. 2018;21(4):271–7.
4. Hollander J, Ranney M, Carr B. No patient left behind: patient-centered healthcare reform. Healthcare Transform. 2016;1(2):114–9. https://doi.org/10.1089/heat.2016.29016.hrc.
5. Gardner MR, Jenkins SM, O'Neil DA, Wood DL, Spurrier BR, Pruthi S. Perceptions of video-based appointments from the patient's home: a patient survey. Telemed J E Health. 2015;21(4):281–5. https://doi.org/10.1089/tmj.2014.0037.

6. Ertel AE, Kaiser T, Shah SA. Using telehealth to enable patient-centered care for liver transplantation. JAMA Surg. 2015;150(7):674–5. https://doi.org/10.1002/lt.24112.3.

7. Zulman DM, Jenchura EC, Cohen DM, Lewis ET, Houston TK, Asch SM. How can eHealth technology address challenges related to multi-morbidity? Perspectives from patients with multiple chronic conditions. J Gen Intern Med. 2015;30(8):1063–70. https://doi.org/10.1007/s11606-015-3222-9.

8. Barnett TE, Chumbler N, Vogel B, Beyth RJ, Qin H, Kobb R. The effective-ness of a care coordination home telehealth program for veterans with dia-betes mellitus: a 2-year follow-up. Am J Manag Care. 2006;12(8):467–74.

9. Aponte-Tinao LA, Farfalli GL, Albergo JI, Plazzotta F, Sommer J, Luna D, de Quirós FGB. Face to face appointment vs. telemedicine in first time appointment orthopedic oncology patients: a cost analysis. Stud Health Technol Inform. 2019;264:512–5. https://doi.org/10.3233/SHTI190275.

10. Prada C, Izquierdo N, Traipe R, Figueroa C. Results of a new telemedi-cine strategy in traumatology and orthopedics. Telemed J E Health. 2019; https://doi.org/10.1089/tmj.2019.0090. [Epub ahead of print]

11. Buvik A, Bergmo TS, Bugge E, Smaabrekke A, Wilsgaard T, Olsen JA. Cost-effectiveness of telemedicine in remote orthopedic consulta-tions: randomized controlled trial. J Med Internet Res. 2019;21(2):e11330. https://doi.org/10.2196/11330.

12. Fenelon C, Murphy EP, Galbraith JG, O'Sullivan ME. Telesurveillance: exploring the use of mobile phone imaging in the follow-up of orthopedic patients with Hand Trauma. Telemed J E Health. 2019;25(12):1244–9. https://doi.org/10.1089/tmj.2018.0210. Epub 2019 Feb 8

13. Ortiz-Piña M, Salas-Fariña Z, Mora-Traverso M, Martín-Martín L, Galiano-Castillo N, García-Montes I, Cantarero-Villanueva I, Fernández-Lao C, Arroyo-Morales M, Mesa-Ruíz A, Castellote-Caballero Y, Salazar-Gravám S, Kronborg L, Martín-Matillas M, Ariza-Vega P. A home-based tele-rehabilitation protocol for patients with hip fracture called @ctive-hip. Res Nurs Health. 2019;42(1):29–38. https://doi.org/10.1002/nur.21922. Epub 2018 Nov 16

14. Buvik A, Bugge E, Knutsen G, Småbrekke A, Wilsgaard T. Patient reported outcomes with remote orthopaedic consultations by telemedicine: a randomised controlled trial. J Telemed Telecare. 2019;25(8):451–9. https://doi.org/10.1177/1357633X18783921. Epub 2018 Jul 4

15. Davidovitch RI, Anoushiravani AA, Feng JE, Chen KK, Karia R, Schwarzkopf R, Iorio R. Home Health services are not required for select total hip arthroplasty candidates: assessment and supplementation with an electronic recovery application. J Arthroplast. 2018;33(7S):S49–55. https://doi.org/10.1016/j.arth.2018.02.048. Epub 2018 Feb 21

16. Chughtai M, Newman JM, Sultan AA, Khlopas A, Navarro SM, Bhave A, Mont MA. The role of virtual rehabilitation in total knee and hip arthro-plasty. Surg Technol Int. 2018;32:299–305.

17. Gilbert AW, Jaggi A, May CR. What is the patient acceptability of real time 1:1 videoconferencing in an orthopaedics setting? A systematic review. Physiotherapy. 2018;104(2):178–86. https://doi.org/10.1016/j.physio.2017.11.217. Epub 2017 Dec 12. Review.

18. Mullen-Fortino M, Rising KL, Duckworth J, Gwynn V, Sites FD, Hollander JE. Presurgical assessment using telemedicine technology: impact on efficiency, effectiveness and patient experience of care. Telemed J E Health. 2018; https://doi.org/10.1089/tmj.2017.0133. [Epub ahead of print]

19. NQF: creating a framework to support measure development for tele-health. Qualityforum.org. Available at: https://www.qualityforum.org/Publications/2017/08/Creating_a_Framework_to_Support_Measure_Development_for_Telehealth.aspx. Published 2017. Accessed 4 Sept 2018.

20. Rising KL, Ricco JC, Printz AD, Woo SH, Hollander JE. Virtual rounds: observational study of a new service connecting family members remotely to inpatient rounds. Gen Int Med Clin Innov. 2016;1(3):50–3.

21. Huigol, YS, Joshi AU, Carr BG, Hollander JE. Giving urban health care access issues the attention they deserve in telemedicine reimbursement policies. Health Affairs Blog. October 12, 2017. Available at: https://www.healthaffairs.org/do/10.1377/hblog20171022.713615/full/. Accessed 4 Sept 2018.

22. Agarwal AK, Gaieski DF, Perman SM, Leary M, Delfin G, Abella BS, Carr BG. Telemedicine REsuscitation and Arrest Trial (TREAT): a feasibility study of real-time provider-to-provider telemedicine for the care of critically ill patients. Heliyon. 2016;2(4):e00099.

23. Powell RE, Henstenburg JM, Cooper G, Hollander JE, Rising KL. Patient perceptions of telehealth primary care video visits. Ann Fam Med. 2017;15(3):225–9.

24. Powell RE, Stone D, Hollander JE. Patient and health system experience with implementation of an enterprise wide telehealth scheduled video visit program: mixed methods study. JMIR Med Inform. 2018, 6(1):e10.p1–7.

25. Papanagnou D, Sicks S, Hollander JE. Training the next generation of care providers: focus on telehealth. Healthcare Transform. 2015;1(1):52–63.

26. Papanagnou D, Stone D, Chandra S, Watts P, Chang AM, Hollander JE. Integrating telehealth emergency department follow up visits into residency training. Cureus. 2018;10(4):e2433.

27. Rising KL, Ward MM, Goldwater JC, Bhagianadh D, Hollander JE. Framework to advance oncology related telehealth. JCO Clin Cancer Inform. 2018; Available at: http://ascopubs.org/doi/pdfdirect/10.1200/CCI.17.00156

28. Glassman DT, Puri AK, Weingarten S, Hollander JE, Stepchin A, Trabulsi E, Gomella LG. A single institution's initial experience with telemedicine. Urology Pract. 2018;5(5):367–71.

29. Nandra K, Koenig G, DelMastro A, Mishler E, Hollander JE, Yeo CJ. Telehealth provides a comprehensive approach to the surgical patient. Am J Surg. 2018; In press. doi: https://doi.org/10.1016/j.amj-surg.2018.09.020. . [Epub ahead of print].
30. Rimer RA, Christopher V, Falck A, et al. Telemedicine in otolaryngology outpatient setting – single center head and neck surgery experience. Laryngoscope. 2018;128(9):2072–5.

Index

© Springer Nature Switzerland AG 2021
A. Atanda Jr., J. F. Lovejoy III (eds.), *Telemedicine in Orthopedic
Surgery and Sports Medicine*,
https://doi.org/10.1007/978-3-030-53879-8

Printed in the United States
By Bookmasters